# Younger Joints Today

## Your 7 Step Plan to turn back the hands of time and get your joints healing, moving and feeling their best

### Dr. Angela Cortal

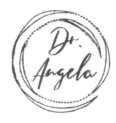

Published by Dr. Angela Cortal ND LLC

PO Box 549, Monmouth, OR 97361

www.drcortal.com

ISBN: PB: 978-1-7353689-0-0; eBook: 978-1-7353689-1-7

Photography by Kristal Passy Photography

Illustrations by Warren Muzak

Graphic design by Desi McAnally

# Table of Contents

# Preface

Hello, congratulations and I see you.

Welcome to Younger Joints Today, my revolutionary approach to anti-aging joint health.

Congratulations on taking the first step in regaining your joint health.

If you have been frustrated with lack of support, lack of options, and feeling dismissed by medical professionals while your joints continue to feel worse and worse by the day, I see you. Because I used to be there, too.

If you have achy joints and feel stuck, this book is for you.

There are many reasons for achy and painful joints.

Osteoarthritis, or degenerative joint disease, is the most common diagnosis related to chronic joint pain. Because it is such a common cause of joint pain, I will be discussing it in-depth in the following chapter, and frequently throughout the rest of the book.

However, if your pain is caused by a spinal disc bulge, meniscus tear, ligament injury, or if it started after menopause or after an accident or injury, my 7

Step Plan can still help. That is because I will be addressing the underlying factors that all these chronic sources of lingering pain have in common.

Use this book to educate yourself on how and why joints degenerate and, more importantly, what you can do to reverse those underlying processes. After the introductory chapter on osteoarthritis, you will find the following chapters each outlining a step of my 7 Step Plan to Younger Joints Today.

Use this book as a self-study tool. As you read, think about what has been investigated in your case. Perhaps some of the topics here have been ignored because someone told you, "It's not relevant." What potential missing pieces are there that could be your next steps in joint healing?

Please feel free to journal as you read through my 7 Step Plan to Younger Joints Today. If you are reading this in print form, you have my explicit blessing to scribble all over this book.

To fully understand the 7 Step Plan, read this book in the order it is written. However, if you would just like to learn about individual topics, dive right into the chapters that interest you most. At the end of each chapter, you will see "The Joint Gist," which are the highlights and the top takeaways of each step.

I have also created the Younger Joints Today Toolkit at www.drcortal.com/toolkit as a partner to this book. To keep the flow and pace of the book's material intact, the Toolkit is where you will find all the additional resources, recipes, meal plans, videos, and ton of other helpful information.

If deep down you know that there's more to your joint pain than just "wear and tear," you're absolutely right. There usually is. Addressing those missing pieces of the puzzle just might be your key to Younger Joints Today.

I wrote this book to provide and equip you with information and education. It is not medical advice, should not be construed as a diagnosis, and is no substitute for medical care. Use the information here to begin a conversation with your healthcare provider. If you are not feeling heard, I encourage you to put together a new care team or seek out a different kind of healthcare. Use this book as your springboard towards better joint health.

Lastly, I would be remiss if I did not discuss the timing of this book's publication in light of the information that follows. I began writing this book long before "viral pandemic" and "quarantine" were household words. I choose not to dwell on our current lifestyle changes (such as my gym being closed at the time of this writing), but instead to focus on the good information that those with chronic joint pain need—regardless of the current events and circumstances. Whether at home or out in the world, aching and painful joints can stop us from living our lives to the fullest. With this in mind, I'd like to share my plan to change that for good and all, starting today.

So, this is how the story begins . . .

. . . and how over the course of the following two decades it developed into my creation of Younger Joints Today, a 7 Step approach informed by research to help thousands reclaim their joints, bodies, and lives.

It all began in 2001 on Mt. Hood in Oregon. I was a young adult, out skiing with friends. While out on the slopes, I carved too close to a snowbank and hit an ice block that was completely hidden in the snow. I came down hard, fast, and at full speed.

After a few startled moments on the ground, my brain started screaming, "OW!" and also, "um, Houston we have a problem. The right leg isn't responding."

I couldn't stand up. I could barely move my right leg at all, which made skiing down out of the question. That day was my first (and hopefully the last) time riding down the hill in the ski patrol rescue sled.

The initial excruciating pain subsided but my right leg remained problematic. A few days later, my leg still wouldn't entirely cooperate. It refused to fully bend or straighten, which meant it was stuck in a sort of a half-bend.

I saw an orthopedic doctor right away. The X-ray showed a likely meniscus tear. The meniscus has the important role of being the shock absorber in the knee. Surgery was scheduled within the week. During the surgery, they found it was actually my knee's anterior cruciate ligament (ACL) which was torn, and not the meniscus.

The tear was surgically corrected, and I was sown up, patched up, and ready to start rehab.

On the surface, I was a "perfectly compliant patient." I did everything I was requested to do to a tee. I took all the medications, attended all the physical therapy appointments, and did all the home exercises.

As the post-operative weeks stretched to months, it was apparent things were still not right.

First, it was knee swelling, causing the return of extreme pain and even a short stint in a wheelchair. Then it was back spasms that were so painful they frequently drove me to tears and on one occasion the emergency room.

The new plan was meds, meds, and more meds.

Opioids: check.

Muscle relaxers: check.

Being told the pain is all in your head: check.

Being told, "you really should be better by now:" check.

I went through it all.

After seeing many providers, over many years, I pieced together for myself how to gain control over the spasms and pain—for the most part.

Years later my atrophied right leg never regained the strength and stability it had pre-injury. Even after a decade, it was still weak and unstable.

I loved attending yoga classes while in medical school. On many occasions I had to carefully stretch my legs out into a pose, placing my "bad leg" down gingerly so that it wouldn't buckle and take me down to the mat.

I had the supposedly corrective surgery.

I was a good patient and did what I was told.

But I was still left with what seemed like a permanent "bad leg."

The joint pain and stiffness that started in my 20s followed me into my 30s. My knee constantly made snap, crackle and pop noises, reminiscent of a particular breakfast cereal.

I was told arthritis is a common aftereffect from knee surgery, but I just couldn't accept that this was happening to me—years earlier than I was prepared to face it. My knee felt as if it were many decades older than my years.

I knew I had to do something about it. I did the only thing I could, which was to become proactive in my joint health in order to reverse the trajectory of my joint pain.

Every aspect of the following 7 Step Plan is based on research. I have pored over countless research articles and textbooks, a fraction of which you will find as references in the bibliography. I can tell you from those many hours of research, you will not find all this information in any one source. Prior to now. The medical textbooks have just not caught up yet, but I hope they do soon. There are millions of Americans suffering from arthritis who are not given the slightest bit of helpful information on what to actually do about it.

Refining this plan has been years in the making. I began my plan with years of research and then experimentation on myself. After that, I brought these therapies and evidence-informed discoveries into my medical practice and have seen nothing short of phenomenal results with my patients. You'll hear several of their stories and testimonies later on, though names and defining characteristics have been modified for confidentiality.

After even more years of developing this approach, myself and my thousands of happy patients serve as living proof that my 7 Step Plan truly does work. These steps are my distillation of the essentials of joint regenerative medicine, informed by research and proven in the clinic.

My joints are now stronger and happier than ever. So are those of so many of my patients. Joints can be happy or unhappy. Just ask anyone experiencing the challenge of living with arthritis.

Before we dive in, I want to initially explain the basics of joint health, disease, and degeneration. In order to understand the root cause of joint pain, we must first start with a little anatomy and physiology. Only after that can we truly understand the reasoning behind my 7 Step Plan to Younger Joints Today.

The causes and factors that influence chronic joint pain are important, because with this knowledge you can then identify and treat the actual underlying causes.

As a Naturopathic Physician, I work from a functional medicine mindset: I try to determine and address the underlying cause of a condition, instead of taking a "Band-Aid" approach which can lead to feeling stuck "managing" chronic joint pain indefinitely. So, let's dive right into understanding arthritis in the following chapter.

# Introduction:

# What is Actually Going on?

It will be enlightening to start with a thorough introduction to all of the little structures that make up our joints. It is essential to understand what may be injured or degenerating, in order to best address and reverse their causes.

Joints allow us to move around. Without joints, you would move like a 5-year old's stick figure drawing. As hilarious as that thought might be, that is exactly how important joints are.

Joints are where two (or more) bones meet. When we talk about joints, we must differentiate between bones and connective tissue. Connective tissue is all the non-bony parts, including joint capsules, ligaments, and tendons (see Figure 1).

Joints move because our brain tells them to. Or more accurately, our brain tells our muscles what to do. Using electrical impulses from our brain through our nervous system, we consciously contract muscles. This causes the contracted muscle to shorten, causing the joint move. We see this as bending, straightening, or rotating (depending on its starting position and orientation of muscle attachments to the bones).

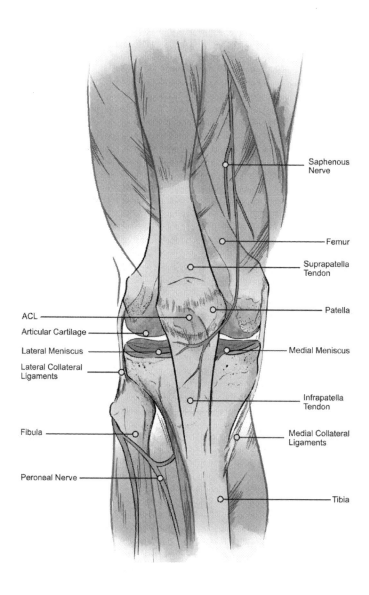

Saphenous
Nerve

Femur

Suprapatella
Tendon

ACL

Patella

Articular Cartilage

Lateral Meniscus

Medial Meniscus

Lateral Collateral
Ligaments

Infrapatella
Tendon

Fibula

Medial Collateral
Ligaments

Peroneal Nerve

Tibia

Figure 1. Knee anatomy. Illustration by Warren Muzak.

Many joints have joint capsules, which like the name suggests, is a flexible structure that surrounds (or encapsulates) the joint. Inside the joint capsule

11

are the cartilage-covered surfaces of the bones where they contact each other.

Cartilage is very dense material covering those bony contact surfaces. Cartilage plays an important role. It is a shock absorber and needs to be very smooth. The intent of the cartilage surfaces is to roll and glide upon one another with the least friction possible (you'll soon see these are key features that change with degeneration).

The joint capsule also contains synovial fluid which is lubrication for the joint.

Tendons are the strong, fibrous connective tissue attaching muscles to bones. Contracting muscles causes tendons to also respond, moving their nearby joints.

Ligaments are similar to tendons but connect bones to bones. The role of ligaments is to provide structural reinforcement for the whole joint complex. They are often on the outer or inner side of the joint to prevent excessive bending or sliding in either direction.

A "joint complex" is used to describe all the bony and connective tissue components of a given joint (knee, or shoulder, for example). This includes the cartilage, joint capsule, ligaments, and tendons surrounding a joint. Some joint complexes are very simple, with just a few structures (like a joint in your pinkie finger). Others are very complex, with many connective tissue structures (like your ankle).

That's enough of anatomy for now. Now let's talk about what happens when joints "go bad."

Joint pain is classified as acute or chronic. The difference is in the timing. Acute joint pain is new, starting within the last few days or weeks. Chronic joint pain is pain that has lasted longer, more than three months. The description itself does not tell you what exactly is going on or why.

Arthritis is a similarly generic description. It just means joint pain (technically joint inflammation). There are many causes of arthritis, such as injuries and trauma, postsurgical, infections, autoimmune, degenerative conditions, and more.

The most common reason for chronic joint pain is degenerative joint disease,[1] also called osteoarthritis. With osteoarthritis, the layer of cartilage over the bones begins to degrade. Healthy cartilage is dense, smooth and absorbs shock. Cartilage affected by osteoarthritis begins to thin, roughen, and become brittle. Sometimes it thins so much that the bone underneath is exposed. The cartilage wearing down can be a cause of pain. On imaging, the cartilage thinning can, at its most severe, be described as "bone on bone" because no more cartilage is seen between the bones (see Figure 2).

Osteoarthritis can affect nearly any joint, but is most common in the knees, hips, hands, neck, and lower back.

The diagnosis is made when someone experiences:[2]

- Chronic, persistent pain in one or more joints
- Morning stiffness, up to 30 minutes

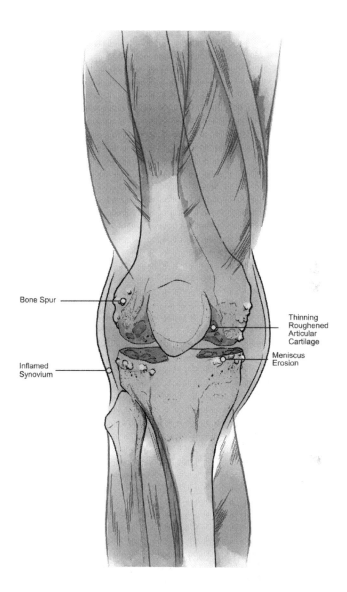

Bone Spur

Thinning Roughened Articular Cartilage

Meniscus Erosion

Inflamed Synovium

Figure 2. Degenerative joint disease of the knee. Illustration by Warren Muzak.

If you experience this and are at least 45 years old, you may not receive any further work-up. There may be many additional physical exam findings (such as joint nodules, deformity, tender joints, and crepitus or a cracking sound when joints move), though all too often those with chronic joint pain do not receive much or any physical exam.

This is such a shame and a huge disservice. How can any proper treatment be recommended without a good physical exam? We need to have an accurate picture of what is going on, in order to strategize what to do next.

An X-ray may be ordered but is not necessary for the doctor to make the diagnosis. This is what is called a clinical diagnosis, because it is based on signs and symptoms, rather than laboratory or imaging findings.

The reason an X-ray is not necessary is that its findings may not correlate with your real-life joint pain, which is the most important aspect. An X-ray may show "advanced" osteoarthritis in someone with little to no pain, or "mild" osteoarthritis in someone who has excruciating, life-altering pain.[3]

Common osteoarthritis findings on X-ray are:[4]

- Joint space narrowing (seen as cartilage degenerates) which, when severe, is described as "bone on bone"
- Osteophytes (bone spurs)
- Cysts and sclerosis (hardening of nearby tissues)

In the US over 54 million adults have osteoarthritis,[5] which is expected to rise to 67 million by 2030.[6] That makes osteoarthritis more common in the US than all current cases of cancer (all types)[7] and diabetes combined.[8] Of course, someone can have more than one diagnosis; this is just to illustrate how very common osteoarthritis is.

Since almost a quarter of all adults in the US have osteoarthritis (23% at the time of this writing to be exact), chances are if you are not experiencing it, you have a friend, family member, or loved one who is. Very likely, you know quite a few folks with the diagnosis.

For such a common condition, not enough is done to change its course.

After being diagnosed, patients are usually recommended exercise, weight loss, and the standard of care treatment which is non-steroidal anti-inflammatory drugs (NSAIDs), such as ibuprofen and referred to physical therapy (PT).

While PT may be great at addressing biomechanical (movement and strength) issues, we now know that there are many systemic health conditions that can bring on and worsen arthritis. This is the basis for many of the following steps in this book.

Physical therapy can be very effective for some, but if someone has one or more non-biomechanical reasons for joint pain, then someone may not adequately respond to care. If the underlying factors are not addressed, they may "fail physical therapy," meaning they have completed a course of treatment with no improvement in their joint pain. If you are working with a physical therapist, I hope that the content of this book helps improve your response to care.

How might this arthritis story end?

You may be one of the those who do not respond well to ibuprofen and PT. Or maybe they help, but temporarily. In the case of ibuprofen, it may even worsen your pain, as the same properties that relieve pain can also work against joint healing. For some they can accelerate the degeneration of arthritis.[9]

Many end up in what is called the "conservative treatment failure gap." This means the conservative treatment (ibuprofen and PT) did not alleviate the pain, but someone is not "bad enough" for a total joint replacement. Or perhaps not a surgical candidate at all.

Many of my patients have been told, "Sorry, there's nothing we can do for you now. Come back in five (or 10) years when it's gotten bad enough. Then we'll replace the joint."

No wonder so many give up and just suffer while the around-the-clock ibuprofen barely makes a dent (and perhaps also causes side effects, such as gastritis).

What about the common recommendations of exercise and weight loss? They are often brought up to those with chronic joint pain, but the conversation is often a woefully inadequate.

If you have been told by your doctor to exercise and lose weight, was there any follow up about what their specific recommendations mean?

What kind of exercise?

How frequently?

For what duration?

What exactly does weight loss do?

And how should it be accomplished?

What is the goal?

It is distinctly unhelpful to be told to exercise and lose weight, and then just move right on to the next topic (or next patient, as it were).

Although weight (measured as body mass index or BMI) may be a risk factor for developing osteoarthritis, it is near-sighted and potentially damaging to focus solely on weight.

We can be confident that it isn't as simple as "your osteoarthritis is due to your BMI." There are a few reasons I say this. One is because not all those with a higher BMI (often categorized as overweight or obese) experience the same level and extent of joint pain.

You may know this from personal experience. Do your left and right joints feel exactly the same? Probably not. But they're all subject to the same bodyweight, right?

If joint pain was only caused by a certain weight, shouldn't they hurt equally? Following this logic, we should expect that every person of the same weight should also have the same level of joint pain.

On the flip side, many thin people experience joint pain. If the whole topic of joint pain were solved with the simple refrain of, "lose weight and exercise," these lower BMI individuals who are physically active should be free of joint pain. I can tell you from personal experience that thin people can (and do) experience crippling joint pain.

Joint pain is not just due to one's BMI. It's not that simple. All we can say is that it's a potential risk factor.

It is just one of many risk factors for osteoarthritis development. You can find many others in any medical textbook on the topic. Most lists will include smoking, occupational factors (such as repetitive stress injuries) and surgical intervention, because a joint that has had surgery is more susceptible to developing arthritis. Additional factors like genetics, gender, and age may also be mentioned.

If you, like me, are not entirely satisfied with this list and feel that there must be more going on beneath the surface, this book was written for you.

I focus on osteoarthritis because it is so prevalent, and very commonly dismissed when seeking care. Those with arthritis often feel defeated and at a loss, and with good reason too. We are offered quick-fix medication "Band-Aids," ultimately surgery, and very little in between.

Although I will be speaking to osteoarthritis throughout this book, this 7 Step Plan can be applied to other degenerative causes of arthritis, arthritis that starts with menopause, and many disc, tendon, and ligament disorders and lingering sports injuries.

All the upcoming topics in this book are vitally important to those with joint pain, but they are often overlooked, disregarded as being important, or just plain ignored. Unlike BMI being checked during a doctor's visit, most of these are never brought up.

If you're thinking that there's got to be a better way, you're right: there is! So let's dive in.

The Joint Gist

- Joints and their cartilage surfaces are vital components affected by arthritis.
- Arthritis is not one specific diagnosis. There are many possible causes.
- Degenerative joint disease is the same as osteoarthritis.
- Osteoarthritis is very common. Roughly 1 out of 4 adults in the US have this diagnosis.
- There are many potential risk factors for the onset and worsening of osteoarthritis. Some are not modifiable, such as gender and age. Some can be, such as whether you smoke or exercise. Many are almost never discussed, such as nutrient and hormone deficiencies.

# STEP 1: Know Your Diagnosis –

# Really Know It

On the surface, it may seem obvious.

I have joint pain because I have arthritis, or a disc bulge or a meniscus tear.

My very first question to you is: how thoroughly have you been evaluated?

My experience as a patient was not uncommon: surgery and medications first, then a course of PT, then more medications.

Over my years in practice, I have lost count of the number of patients with chronic pain who report they have never received a hands-on physical exam from a previous healthcare provider.

Jenny was a prime example of this. She's a lovely 45-year old woman who experienced chronic back pain starting with a roll-over car accident five years prior.

She had "tried everything" through a large local medical establishment. She "failed" conservative treatment, meaning that over the counter pain relievers, a course of PT and steroid injections (another common treatment) did not improve her pain.

She had gotten imaging (X-rays then an MRI), but the findings only revealed arthritis in her low back, a common finding.

She was told she was not a surgical candidate so was out of treatment options. She felt ready to give up hope and felt far older than her 45 years. But (a very important but!) I quickly figured out that she had never had a thorough physical exam.

That's right . . . all the years of being bounced around from doctor to doctor. Every kind of pain specialist. No physical exam. It's such a shame. This should not happen, but I hear it all the time.

If you are going to a doctor for pain, at a bare minimum you should receive a physical exam. I don't think that's a radical view.

That is where Step 1 begins: a comprehensive physical exam.

Pain can (and does) come from joint disease but can also come from many other types of tissue such as a ligament, tendon, meniscus, or nerve—to name a few. It is important to assess all structures around a site of chronic pain, as these are very often overlooked.

If you have chronic joint pain, you need to be thoroughly assessed. Otherwise, an important part of the picture is almost certainly missing.

This just makes sense. With degeneration, over time there can also be compensations, including changes in muscle engagement, positioning of the joint at rest and during motion. The whole way in which a joint moves (or doesn't move) is altered. This will cause ripple effects through the joint complex affecting far more than just a "loss of cartilage" we can see on an X-ray.

Very often I find far more than "just the joint" is responsible for someone's entire pain picture.

In reality, that is what pain is like: a picture with different colors, textures, a background and a foreground. Chronic pain is rarely one dimensional. It very often is complex and layered.

We can't treat what we don't identify. That is why it is so important to start with a professional who will provide you with an in-depth physical evaluation. Only with the whole picture can you get the most accurate plan on your next steps.

### How important is imaging?

Imaging such as X-rays and MRIs can provide good information. Often they do not tell the whole story (like in Jenny's case), and sometimes they tell the wrong story. That is, their findings do not always correlate with pain.

A good example of this is degenerative disc disease, which is similar to osteoarthritis, but affects spinal discs. When someone experiences chronic low back pain, their doctor may order an X-ray and perhaps also an MRI. If disc generation is found on the imaging, it is often quickly chalked up as the cause of the low back pain—perhaps with no correlating physical exam. Just because disc degeneration is found on an image, we cannot say it is definitively causing the pain.

Research shows this to be the case. In looking at X-rays and MRIs of people with no back pain (asymptomatic individuals), we see disc degeneration in 37% of 20-year olds, increasing by age up to 96% of 80-year olds.[10] We see similar findings with disc bulging and protrusion. Not every degenerated disc, bulge, and protrusion seen on imaging causes pain.

Sometimes, the wrong story gets told if the imaging picks up on a common finding that has nothing to do with your pain. As we age, the majority of us have what we would call incidental findings. The report may say something that sounds scary but is actually very commonplace (and may not be the true source of pain), such as minor disc bulges and arthrosis of joints.

While imaging is less likely to miss a fracture or dislocation, it may not find minor tears and may miss pain resulting from dysfunctional movement or weak tissues. Those kinds of pathology may not be seen on imaging.

Which brings me back to Jenny. At our first appointment, we started with a comprehensive physical exam. She needed to start at Step 1. What we found surprised her.

Upon the physical exam, we found many sources of her pain that had never been identified before, including ligaments surrounding her sacroiliac joints (they hold the pelvic bones to the sacrum down near your back pockets) and lumbar stabilizing ligaments.

We found many sites of ligament weakness, instability, and pain that hid from her X-rays and MRIs. These structures have the very important job of keeping the lower spine and sacrum stable and connected. Likely due to a past injury, they were not doing their job.

During that first appointment, we were able to get further into investigating Jenny's source of pain than she had gotten in the prior five years. All because she had been given one recommendation after another, without anyone actually performing a comprehensive physical exam.

A thorough evaluation dictates how the rest of the story unfolds. Pain originating from damaged ligaments is handled differently than pain coming from inflamed nerves. Once we know what we're working with, where the pain is really coming from, then we can put together the best path forward.

STEP 1: Know Your Diagnosis

The Joint Gist

- There are many sources of pain. Even if you have an arthritis diagnosis, you can still have pain stemming from injured ligaments, tendons, nerves, fascia, and other connective tissue.
- If you have not received a thorough physical exam, find a doctor who will provide you with this essential analysis. You deserve it.
- Imaging may be helpful but may not show where your pain is actually coming from.

# STEP 2: Eat to Heal Your Joints

You are what you eat. We all are. Even Sarah, a stubborn and vibrant attorney who is 53 years young. She started seeing me in 2017, and we got on the same page some time in 2019. One big sticking point was diet. Specifically, her dieting.

I hate the word "diet." It will appear many times in this chapter out of necessity in using a word to describe what we choose to eat . . . but I still hate it.

People use the word "diet" in many unhealthy ways. It often involves severe restriction, and many times, there are unhealthy motives behind dieting and diets.

Instead of "diet" meaning "restriction," I prefer these definitions instead: "habitual nourishment" and "regimen of intent." How do you intend to nourish yourself every day? Now that is a mindset I can get behind.

Sarah was one of the millions of women who had been compulsively tracking and analyzing all her food, based on guidelines from her diet tracking app. On the surface, her diet appeared healthy. It included green smoothies, organic food, and plenty of water. But upon closer examination, sticking to her calorie count goal left her with key nutritional deficiencies that stood in the way of healing her chronically achy knees, shoulder, wrists, and hands.

What's the best diet? I believe it is that which supports your health, your joints, and all the rest of you. Starting with a foundation of nutrition, focused on what your joints need to reduce inflammation and regenerate is where we will begin.

The standard American diet (SAD) is the starting point for many, and it is rife with problems. Millions of Americans are unintentionally eating a diet based in over-processed, nutrient-poor, which fuels many chronic diseases such as obesity, diabetes, high blood pressure, kidney disease, and dementia.

The majority of US adults (perhaps now up to 87.8%[11]) have at least one component of metabolic syndrome, a constellation of health conditions which increase the risk for chronic diseases such as those mentioned above.

The diagnosis for metabolic syndrome requires having three or more of the following:[12]

- Impaired fasting glucose (100 mg/dL or higher) or impaired oral glucose tolerance test
- High blood pressure (130/85 mm Hg or higher)
- Elevated fasting triglycerides (150 mg/dL or higher)
- Low HDL cholesterol (less than 40 mg/dL in men or less than 50 mg/dL in women)
- Abdominal obesity (waist circumference of more than 102 cm in men or more than 88 cm in women)

Let's pause for a moment. Why am I talking about metabolic disease in a book about joints? Because it impacts chronic joint disease, plain and simple. They are closely linked.

The SAD contributes to insulin resistance and nutrient deficiencies. Both of these set the stage for an earlier onset and worsening of arthritis.

If you are one of the millions of Americans that fit the criteria of metabolic syndrome, you most likely have insulin resistance. This can be evaluated by your doctor.

Insulin resistance is a hormonal imbalance that creates and worsens high blood sugar levels. As you will later see, it also creates a whole host of other issues relevant to joint health and disease.

At the most basic level, insulin resistance is an inefficiency in the glucose-insulin regulation system. Glucose is a form of sugar that provides energy to our cells. It is a component of many sugars and carbohydrates and is released from these foods during digestion. Then they circulate in the body to provide a source of energy to our cells. Insulin is the hormone produced by the pancreas that tells the glucose what to do and where to go.

If all is operating well between glucose and insulin, we call that insulin sensitivity. The right amount of insulin is produced and directs the glucose to appropriately enter the cells, tissues, and organs that need more fuel or energy.

Insulin sensitivity and insulin resistance fall on a spectrum. The more efficient the signaling, the more *sensitive*. The more inefficient the signaling, the more *resistant*.

We see this inefficiency, or resistance, crop up in several ways. As insulin resistance develops, more and more insulin is required from the pancreas in order to direct the same amount of energy (glucose) into the cells. As the glucose is waiting to get into the cells, it is sitting in the bloodstream, which we see as high blood sugar levels.

We know that high blood sugar over time is dangerous, apparent from diabetic complications such as neurologic, kidney, retinal, and cardiovascular disease.

Our body has an inherent wisdom and is always trying to help us the best it can. In order to respond to this high blood sugar, compensation mechanisms kick in. These include storing excess glucose in the liver (which can then lead to nonalcoholic fatty liver disease) and releasing yet more and more insulin into the bloodstream to try and deal with the high blood sugar.

What we see over time is that insulin resistance creates its own snowball effect between glucose, insulin, and insulin receptors, leading to greater and greater glucose spikes. This then leads to more insulin being released, with many health complications seen as possible fallout effects.

At its core, insulin resistance is a hormonal dysfunction, not a specific disease. It underlies many chronic diseases such as weight gain, fatigue, hypertension, kidney dysfunction, heart disease, elevated cholesterol, and also arthritis.

Insulin is a common denominator between food, physiology, and joint health. When present, excess insulin creates an inflammatory response within the joints and is a major contributor to the appearance and worsening of arthritis.

Seven out of eight US adults have at least one marker of metabolic syndrome,[13] which is not enough to get the diagnosis label (remember, you need three), but enough for us to pay attention. If you have been diagnosed with osteoarthritis, there is a good chance that you may be one of those with a marker of metabolic disease present.

The question is . . . now, what do we do?

29

We first look at where it all begins. Since the dietary components are the original fuel to the fire of this glucose and insulin excess spiraling effect, addressing these is where we start.

Looking at food, we will start with understanding the macronutrients. Macronutrients are the types of calories (energy) that we get from food and include protein, fat, and carbohydrates.

In the case of insulin resistance, we need to reduce the amount of fuel feeding fire, which triggers joint inflammation. One way we can do this is by altering the components of our daily meals, thereby addressing the irritation happening inside of our joints due to excess insulin.

The key aspects to focus on when it comes to research looking at nutrition and joint health are:

- Consuming healthy, non-processed forms of fat and protein
- Getting adequate levels of protein
- Minimizing simple and refined carbohydrates
- Avoiding added and hidden sources of sugars

We can work to reverse insulin resistance (if it is present), thereby reducing inflammation and providing the building blocks you need to build up your joints.

### Fats

Fat has long been vilified as a dangerous poison that will make us sick, overweight, and unhealthy. We now know that that was an extreme over-simplification and that unprocessed forms of fats are necessary for well-rounded nutrition. When it comes to joint health, the source and quality matter, not the fat calories.

Foods that are nutritional and naturally high in fat include many types of grass-fed or pastured meat, fish and seafood, avocado, coconut, nuts, seeds, olive oil, and other unrefined plant oils. Many processed foods, such as fast food, may be high in fat as well, but they are not perceived as the same in your body.

Your body recognizes all the components of your diet and responds differently to each dietary building blocks. Some nourish and support health, some undermine it; particularly when eaten in excess.

Food is communication. What are you telling your body? Tell your body that you are supporting it by incorporating plenty of whole and unprocessed sources of proteins and fats.

We all need adequate dietary fat intake in order to make the appropriate amount of hormones. Hormones (as you will see in Step 5) require fat since fat compounds are what makes up their molecular backbone. Give your body what it needs by starting with nutrition first.

Foods high in fat comprise a wide spectrum of healthful components. Some types of fat can be particularly beneficial for joint health and include monounsaturated fatty acids (MUFAs) and polyunsaturated fatty acids (PUFAs).

MUFAs are found in minimally refined plant oils such as olive oil and sesame oil. Incorporating them into your diet may lower inflammation associated with arthritis. This has been shown in animal models,[14] so now we need human studies. Sign me up, yum!

PUFAs, such as omega-3 fatty acids, are found in wild-caught salmon but are also present in grass-fed beef. You will read more about PUFAs used as a supplement in Step 6.

Quality counts! We can actually see that people eating grass-fed beef have higher PUFAs[15] in their bloodstream than those eating beef fed corn and grains. Higher dietary levels of PUFAs are associated with slowing the arthritis process (reduced loss of knee cartilage[16]). You can make sure your diet has adequate PUFAs by regularly including fish, seafood, and grass-fed or pastured meat in your meals.

### Protein

We need protein to heal. Whether the joint pain is acute (a few weeks ago) or chronic (lingering for months or years), adequate protein is essential in order to heal. Damaged joints, ligaments, and tendons need sufficient protein to rebuild themselves.

A 2016 study in the British Journal of Nutrition[17] found that women in their 60s and 70s who had higher protein intake had better physical function than women who had moderate or low protein intake. They were stronger and had a better physical performance.

What exactly counts as high protein? In this study, it was defined as 1.2 grams of protein per kilogram of body weight (g/kg), which works out to at least 73 grams of protein for a woman weighing 61 kg (135 lbs).

In the US, the Recommended Dietary Allowance (RDA) of protein for adults is 0.8 g/kg, which is two-thirds of the "high protein intake" mentioned above. The RDA guidance is based on preventing pathologic deficiencies. This means that below 0.8g/kg, people experience disease relating to protein deficiency. I don't know about you, but that's not good enough for me. The 1.2 g/kg above indicates more optimal levels of protein intake for healing, strength and recovery, not just the minimum needed to not waste away.

For those with osteoarthritis, we know that low protein intake is associated with less strength.[18] With chronic joint pain, we need all the strength we can get to support healthy joint function.

Many people exist long-term in a state of mild protein deficiency. They may not notice any particular ill effect at all. The only sign may be a lingering achy pain that just doesn't seem to heal.

In my experience, many of my female patients under eat when it comes to protein, many not even meeting that meager 0.8 g/kg level.

Daily intake is not something you can easily guess by looking at your food. You can work with a nutritional professional who can help analyze this or get a rough estimate from a diet tracking app.

I have seen long-term use of these diet apps be a major contributor towards deprivation and unhealthy eating patterns (along with them often setting unhealthy calorie deficiency goals). So if you use one of these to assess your protein intake, I recommend their use with caution. Their best use is to track a few average days, take a look at the calculations, then use that information to guide your best judgment going forward.

I am not focusing on calories. I am not talking about calorie restriction. I am wanting you to eat enough protein on a daily basis. Depending on your body weight and goals (building muscle, repairing connective tissue), a daily goal amount may be 75-100 grams of protein. As with all information in this book, run this by your doctor, especially if you have certain medical conditions such as chronic kidney disease.

If you have read high protein is bad for your bones, I want to dispel that myth right now. For those who have a low bone mineral density (osteopenia and osteoporosis), eating enough protein is actually very important and has been shown to improve bone density.[19]

So, let's all make sure we are getting enough protein in our diet.

## Carbohydrates

The last macronutrient to discuss is carbohydrates. This form of energy comes from many types of food sources and comprises the majority of the fuel source in foods such as grains (such as wheat, rice, barley, and oats), beans, corn, and root vegetables (such as potatoes, sweet potatoes, and beets).

At its foundation, carbohydrates come from sugars (such as glucose) that get broken down in the digestive tract. Sometimes it's obvious what contains sugar, such as candy or soda pop. Sometimes it is more hidden, such as in dressings, sauces, and beverages that may contain added sugar.

With metabolic disease being extremely common and a triggering factor for arthritis, it is helpful to be aware of all the potential sources of sugar in our diet.

Instead of sugar, the recipes in the appendix use monk fruit and erythritol as sweeteners for those recipes where a sweet taste is expected. In general, it is wise to keep sweeteners minimal in your diet. For the occasional low-sugar sweet, monk fruit and erythritol appear to be good options for many.

## Fruits and vegetables

The dietary composition of fruits and vegetables is highly variable. We already mentioned that root vegetables are very carbohydrate-dense. I call all the other non-root vegetables "above-ground vegetables," just to keep things simple. These tend to be more fiber-rich than carbohydrate-dense vegetables, so are good choices for those with metabolic and arthritis concerns.

A few examples of these are broccoli, kale, and cucumbers. They all grow above ground and are rich in fiber but lower in carbohydrates compared to root vegetables.

Dairy such as milk, cream, butter, and cheese are variable in their macronutrient content. Some are mostly carbohydrate, such as milk (particularly low-fat milk). Others are primarily fat, such as butter and cream. As with meat products, grass-fed sources will contain more healthful fats. If you tolerate dairy products, those that are richer in protein and fat can be an acceptable component of meals from a metabolic and joint health standpoint.

You will find an example shopping list and meal plan in the Younger Joints Today Toolkit, at www.drcortal.com/toolkit, along with my home kitchen-tested recipes in US and metric units.

Approach this by taking a look at what your current meal is (or what you're planning to cook) and think about what you may want to adjust in terms of its macronutrient ratio and thus nutritional building blocks.

Focus on those foods that are whole quality sources of fat and protein in order to crowd out those that contain just refined carbohydrates.

We are looking to find a nutritional balance that works best for you and your joints long term, so I like to take a balanced approach. Some examples include adding more meat, nuts, seeds, and olive oil to your salad. Or making a salad instead of mashed potatoes. Add more fibrous vegetables to your meal. Take a smaller scoop of rice or beans. Keep repeating and refining the process, learning and adjusting as you go.

We are seeking to include more of the macronutrients that contain building blocks to support rebuilding joints and minimize those that do not help.

Collagen

This compound is very important in the creation and maintenance of healthy joints and chances are you get very little of it in your diet.

Collagen is the primary building block of joints, ligaments, and tendons. That means you need to be making sufficient collagen in order to create new cartilage, ligament, and tendon tissue.[20] Consuming collagen is an efficient way to guarantee you have enough of these building blocks on hand for regeneration.

Food sources of collagen are animal-derived, from sources where collagen is concentrated in their tissues, such as joints, ligaments, and tendons. There is no plant-based source of collagen, though plant-derived precursors do exist.

Have you ever cooked a broth, fish, or meat dish and had a layer of gelatin coagulate on the top? That is mostly collagen. Without conscious effort, most of us may not regularly consume collagen-rich foods. I would like to change that.

In the appendix, you will find my favorite ways to easily incorporate this nutrient into your diet, such as my Kitchen Sink Bone Broth, warming and hearty Oxtail Soup recipe or even as a dessert such as my Key Lime Pie Parfait. These are just a few ideas that have been kitchen-tested and doctor-approved. Create your own collagen-rich recipes and let me know what you come up with.

Your body is working hard to regenerate and heal each and every day. Give it all the building blocks it needs, which includes collagen, on a daily basis.

Step 6 covers supplementation, and collagen will make an appearance there too. If getting a serving of collagen-rich foods in your diet every single day is too challenging, adding in a collagen supplement can be a good alternative. Skip ahead to Step 6 now if you want to know what to look for (and what to avoid) when selecting collagen supplements.

Collagen recipes and supplementation was my way to make inroads with Sarah. Eat fat? No way. Her mindset was firmly stuck in the fat-phobic 80s era. Because of calorie counting, she was very restrictive with her protein intake too. And while green smoothies and salads can certainly be part of a healthy diet, on their own they just weren't enough for her to heal.

While she was very (very) slowly warming to the idea of grass-fed and pastured sources of fat and protein in her diet, we started first with the addition of collagen, such as bone broth and supplementation.

Within a month she noticed a radical change. She wasn't waking up with the same level of morning stiffness. She could now get down her stairs with ease. Not only did Sarah notice much less stiffness and achiness, but she also noticed improved strength and was now progressing further than ever before in her weight training class. We slowly and steadily built her back up from her years of deprivation and deficiency.

## Putting this all together

Think about your food in terms of, "What is it mostly? Protein, fat, or carbohydrates?" I want you to understand what your food is made of, in order to make the best nutritional choices for your needs.

Include on a daily basis:

- One to three servings per day of foods that are rich in healthy fat, such as pasture-raised meat, fish, seafood, avocado, coconut, olive oil, butter, eggs, nuts, and seeds.
- Three servings per day of foods that are rich in protein, such as meat and eggs. These can be the same as above. Find a variety of fat- and protein-rich foods that you enjoy eating.
- One serving per day of collagen-rich foods or supplementation, discussed in Step 6.
- De-emphasize foods that are mostly just made of refined carbohydrates, such as wheat, rice, barley, oats, beans, corn, and root vegetables.
- Minimize added sugars, such as those found in sweets, desserts, and soda pop.
- Avoid dehydration by drinking at least 64 ounces of water daily. This keeps our cartilage as plump as possible.

What is this diet anyway? Gluten-free? Low-carb? Paleo? Keto?

While there can be many beneficial aspects to all these approaches, we are not necessarily following any particular "name brand" diet.

This plan uses nutrition as a medical intervention, so is evidence-informed as to what we need to rebuild joints.

"Food as medicine" is a foundational piece of a functional medicine plan. Our approach here is to use specific foods for their key components, our building blocks to future healthy joints.

If you want to support good physical health with your diet, make sure to incorporate all the vital aspects your body needs.

This is also (and specifically) *not* a weight loss diet. If you have insulin resistance, you may notice some weight loss as this process slows and reverses. But this is by no means a weight loss diet. That is not our focus. My real goal is to support achieving your healthiest, strongest, and most capable version of yourself, for as long as possible.

STEP 1: Know Your Diagnosis

STEP 2: Eat to Heal Your Joints

The Joint Gist

- Metabolic disease is very common and contributes to the appearance and worsening of heart disease, diabetes, and arthritis.
- Excess insulin appears to be one of the common denominators regarding connection to arthritis.

- Adequate nutrition for joint health includes natural (unprocessed) fats, particularly those containing omega-3 fatty acids, as well as protein and collagen.
- Collagen is a major building block of joints, cartilage, and other connective tissue. It is often deficient in our diet.
- Foods containing processed and added sugars should be minimized as much as possible.

# STEP 3: Move and Strengthen Your Joints

If you intend to improve your joint function, you need to get moving and stay moving. A sedentary lifestyle spells poor nutrition and poor oxygenation for your joints and connective tissue.

If you never challenge your body, it will grow (or remain) weak. That may sound obvious, but this holds true whether the whole body or one specific joint.

Just like muscles will wither after weeks in a cast, being sedentary is like casting your whole body. I know that if you're in chronic pain, you may not feel like exercising. Everything hurts, and you don't have the energy for it.

I get it. I've been there. But you can't remain there if you hope to change your trajectory. We have to get you moving. We start with what you can do and go from there.

This was a big sticking point with Sharon. Her knees and ankles were in near-constant pain. She had been diagnosed with mild osteoarthritis in both knees right after her 50th birthday, which had continued to worsen over the intervening decade. Adding to that, for the last several years her ankles started to constantly ache as well.

Like so many, she had a sedentary desk job, working for the county. She sat all day, every day, and was too tired to do much of anything on evenings and weekends. She was stuck in a sedentary loop. Lack of exercise creates more fatigue, which then means zero motivation to exercise. On and on it goes.

Muscle strength is vitally important when addressing joint pain. Sarcopenia is the medical term for muscle wasting and is strongly associated with degenerative joint disease, as well as earlier death and disability.

Without a conscious effort to reverse it, this muscle wasting begins in the 3rd decade of life and continues throughout, accelerating during our later decades of life.

A doctor can determine if you have sarcopenia, but here is a rough guide. If you are in your 30s or 40s (or older), and have paid no attention to developing physical capacity, performance and strength during your adult years, you likely have some degree of sarcopenia.

Exercise is necessary to address chronic joint pain. The research on this is compelling. Many types of exercise have been shown to improve joint pain. Walking, stretching, aerobic fitness classes, isometric exercise, balance exercise, core exercise, Pilates, yoga, aquatic exercise, and strength training are among those that have been proven to improve pain levels and function for those with chronic joint pain.[21,22,23]

If the thought of "doing exercise" makes you cringe, be creative and find an enjoyable way to move your body. If you're just starting out, pick an activity that you like and that feels good. Maybe that means finding a dance class with fun music, being active outdoors, or taking a water aerobics class.

The key is to approach it with receptivity. If you resent your time being active, that will build long-term negative, so let's work creatively to prevent that.

Once you get moving, then focus on adjustments specific to your joint needs. But as a starting point, just start somewhere.

If local and online fitness offerings are not appealing to you (at first), take a look at the countless fitness apps and videos available to get you started. There are many creative apps that help you be active such as running from zombies (Zombies, Run!) or saving all of humanity as a superhero (Superhero Workout).

This was how we first sneaked exercise into Sharon's routine. After being introduced to a kids' yoga app by her grandchildren, Sharon started using it each morning before work.

Sure, it might be created for children, but who's to judge? Movement is movement. From there, she then felt comfortable getting into fitness classes and most recently has started working with a local trainer I referred her to.

Start where you need to start. I mean it. If you are new to adding physical movement into your life, don't start too hard too fast. That is a recipe for emotional defeat or potential injury.

Instead, start with gentle movement such as walking, water aerobics, yoga, Tai Chi, or Qi Gong. Look into in-person or virtual group classes taught by your local gym, fitness center, or community center. Many have options where you can participate in a seated position if you need it. It may suit your needs to work with a trainer that specializes in return to activity.

Ease your way into physical challenges. Get familiar with what is "easy" for you, then carefully progress to more challenging positions or holding poses for longer. For example, a plank position can feel very easy for 5 seconds but challenging after a minute or more.

That was how I began my road to physical recovery. First yoga classes, then a few more fitness classes. I went from not being able to do a single squat without knee pain and instability to now years later being able to do squats, deadlifts and other weight lifting using weights as heavy as I am. That did not happen overnight. It was a steady development over years, with expert guidance every step of the way.

Find the progressions or increasing challenges that are right for you by working with a movement professional or trainer. After you are comfortable with mobilization and positions, then move on to challenging strength and resistance.

Begin by focusing on improving range of motion, specific to your joints. Whether we are talking about knees, hips, low back, or other joints, each has their own range of motion, or the ability to flex, extend, and rotate.

Gentle stretching is one way to warm up the joint. Depending on which joint we are focusing on, we want to introduce flexion, extension, and/or rotation by exploring "the corners" or the end range of the joint. Be cautious to not overly force a joint. We just want to play with its movement pattern without forcing anything or creating excess pressure.

As you move and stretch, take a moment to check in. Is it comfortable? Does it hurt? Does it feel "not right?" Stretching should feel comfortable.

If you are already experiencing some joint pain prior to exercise, then that may continue while you are exercising. We expect that. I encourage you to move even if you experience ongoing joint pain. However, exercise should not cause or increase pain. That is a sign that it needs to be carefully addressed and modified for you.

We simply cannot wait for your joint pain to completely disappear before you start exercising. It just doesn't work that way.

It is safe and recommended for those with arthritis to exercise. You just have to find what works best for you. Exercise improves joint pain. Avoiding exercise worsens joint pain.

Even if you start with a kids' yoga app, it doesn't matter. What matters is reversing years or decades of inactivity. Starting today. Start small, then build. Sharon is now doing great because she was not only able to find the exercise that worked for her (and that she enjoyed), she was able to use it as a foundation to get her knee and ankle pain completely under control.

Be sure to get guidance when you are first starting out, any time any pain arises, and when you're ready to add resistance or strength training. Don't avoid coaching; embrace this step. It means you're ready to invest in getting strong. You are taking your joint health seriously.

The following are range of motion and stretching activities, with the key joints being addressed below. These are general ideas and starting places, which should be individualized and ultimately guided and coached to fit your needs.

The order of progression for any joint starts with range of motion and stretching to understand its movement pattern, such as how much it can bend and rotate. Then we add on isometric and bodyweight exercises, which challenge the joints using gravity.

Begin with gentle activity, such as walking and stretching. For most people, 30 minutes three times per week is a great starting place. You may then work

that up to 5-7 times per week. When you are ready, add in resistance and strengthening exercise to reverse muscle wasting, develop joint strength and ultimately improve joint pain. But don't overdo it. You can alternate your gentle activity days with your strength training days.  For those looking to use functional movement to address joint pain,
starting with 30 minutes of resistance exercise three times per week is a good first step.


Though I encourage you to work with a professional, the following are just a few of the many exercises that can be done at home with no specialized equipment. Here I am, doing these activities at home. I welcome you to join me from the comfort of your home. Some focus on joint mobility, others muscle activation and resistance. I welcome you to try those that best fit your needs.

Focusing on knee mobility and activation:

# Stepping Over/Under

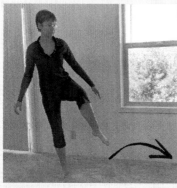

- Step sideways, pretending there are obstacles to step over and duck under.
- As you step down with the leading leg, duck your head and upper body at least a foot down and back up.

- Take 3-5 steps in this manner then repeat in the other direction.
- Repeat a total of 3-5 times.

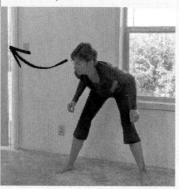

# Squat

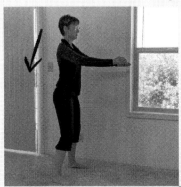

- Place feet shoulder-width apart, facing forward.
- Bend your knees as you lower down towards the floor.
- Hold onto a counter or table in front if needed for balance.

- Keep your weight centered.
- Return to a standing position by pressing through your heels.
- Repeat a 12 times.

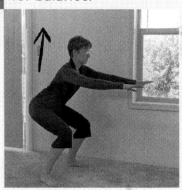

Focusing on hip and low back mobility and activation:

# Hip Windshield wipers

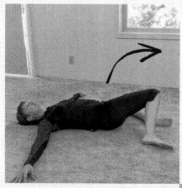

- Lay on your back, knees bent and feet on the ground, hip-width apart.
- Rest your arms straight out from your body.
- Let your knees both fall to one side, stopping before you feel the hip of the opposite side raising.

- Use your lower core and trunk to return your legs to neutral.
- Repeat 12 times on each side.

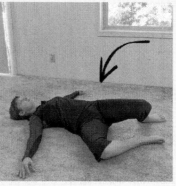

# Hip Hinge

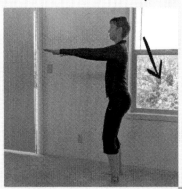

- Place feet shoulder-width apart, facing forward.
- Option to stand with back a foot away from the wall.
- Bend at the hips, keeping back in a neutral (not bent) position.

- If near a wall, your rear will contact the wall.
- The glutes and lower trunk should feel active.
- Return to a standing position by pressing through your heels.
- Repeat a 12 times.

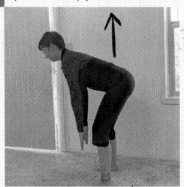

# Bird Dog

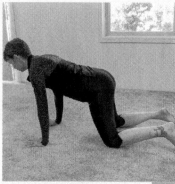

- Start "on all fours" with hands and knees on the ground.
- Activate your core and press your left leg behind you, aiming for your leg to be parellel to the ground.

- Lift your right arm up to parallel with the ground.
- Option: moving just an arm then just a leg.
- Hold position 5 seconds and repeat 3-5 times each side.

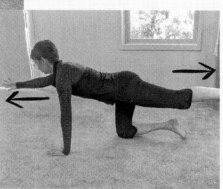

# Dead Bug

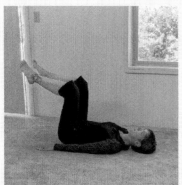

- Lay on your back, arms at your side, knees bent and feet flat on the ground.
- Activate your core to lift your left leg up so your shin is parallel to the ground.

- At the same time, lift your right arm up and over your head.
- Go slow, taking 10-20 seconds to complete.
- Repeat 3-5 times on each side.

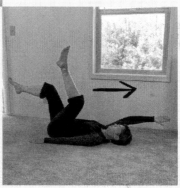

# Plank

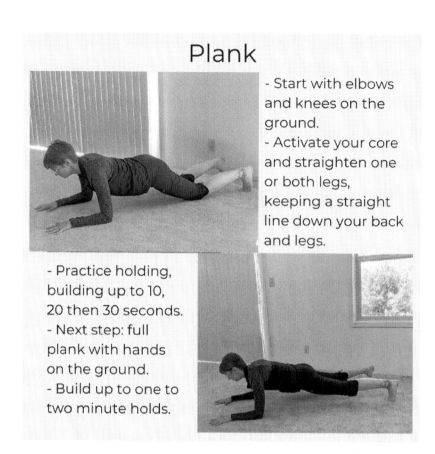

- Start with elbows and knees on the ground.
- Activate your core and straighten one or both legs, keeping a straight line down your back and legs.

- Practice holding, building up to 10, 20 then 30 seconds.
- Next step: full plank with hands on the ground.
- Build up to one to two minute holds.

Exercise demonstration video links, where I am coached through these by a professional, are included in the Younger Joints Today Toolkit at www.drcortal.com/toolkit.

Moving from gentle activity to resistance exercises increases joint stability and strength, and should be guided by a professional. It is very possible to injure yourself with poor form or using too much weight. Enter strength training with the mindset that investing in professional guidance will be extremely beneficial for your joint health.

When you start strength training, you will also get an added health bonus. There is a positive feedback effect between healthy developed muscles and hormones, such as testosterone and estrogen. This interplay creates a positive healing response for our muscles, joints, and tendons. We will dive further into the connection between hormones and joint health in Step 5.

In addition to testosterone and estrogen benefits, strength training specifically in older adults reverses insulin resistance (an important health concern described in the last chapter) as it improves knee arthritis pain and joint function.[24]

Get moving, then get strong. Your hormones will thank you, and you'll be taking the most potent anti-aging medicine there is.

As strength develops, so does grip strength specifically. We know that grip strength is inversely associated with mortality,[25] which means the stronger your grip, the longer your lifespan. And that's something we can all get behind.

STEP 1: Know Your Diagnosis

STEP 2: Eat to Heal Your Joints

STEP 3: Move and Strengthen Your Joints for Recovery

The Joint Gist

- Get moving
- Stay moving

- Get strong
- Keep getting stronger
- Have fun!

# STEP 4: Leveraging Lifestyle Medicine

This chapter begins with Jan's story. Jan came to me for nagging hip pain. Her hips had been bothering her for as long as she could remember, making her feel much older than her 48 years. After seeing what her mother went through following hip replacement surgery, Jan adamantly refused to consider surgery though she had been told it was her last and only option.

For Jan, we improved her hip by addressing factors such as her mindset and habits. Jan managed an upscale bar in town, which meant long hours on her feet, irregular and late hours as well as a significant alcohol intake. Though we couldn't do much to about her work duties, we decided to address the lifestyle factors that were directly working against her, namely her drinking habit.

In this chapter, we take a deep dive into all things concerning mindset and lifestyle medicine. Healthy habits such as regular exercise and good nutrition will only take you so far if you're not in the right mindset. Lifestyle habits, as you will see, can work for you or against you, despite your best efforts to address other steps to joint health.

Let's start with identifying where your mindset is at. It is a spectrum, where on one end is a fixed mindset and on the other end is a growth mindset (credit: psychologist Carol Dweck).[26]

The fixed mindset tells us, "This is the way it is. This is the way it will always be. Change is hard. It's not worth it. I probably can't even do it anyway."

Have you heard this before? How about in regard to joint pain? I know I have. I was guilty of saying it to myself many times in the past. Those times are over for me. They had to be. I could never have gotten better being in a fixed mindset. It's difficult to change the course of nearly any chronic disease while in a fixed mindset.

On the other end is the growth mindset. The growth mindset says, "Change is possible. Challenges are worth it. Take a big-picture view. I am worth what it takes to get to where I want to go."

As you read through this chapter and this book, here are some journaling prompts to reflect upon:

What do you want to change?

Why do you want to change?

What in your life has become unacceptable?

What is joint pain preventing you from doing in your life?

What would change look like?

What would you need to accomplish it?

What tools do you need? Where would you get them from?

Who is on your support team?

Are there missing roles to fill on this team?

What fears are coming up?

Do you believe you're worth it?

Is your future worth it?

Be open, flow with your processing. There are no right answers, and your answers will invariably change day-to-day. We are just starting to get a sense of the mindset and intentions behind what we do, what we don't do, and why.

We are all doing the best we can. Always. Whatever you think of as a "bad habit" is the best you came up with to serve its purpose. Very often, it is an unconscious choice. Whether the original trigger was stress, anxiety, trauma, fear, lack of security, boredom, or something else, our habits are triggered by cues, both internal and external.

Habits serve a purpose. They are meeting the need of that original trigger. That doesn't mean they can't be analyzed and improved, if we wish to do that. We first start by taking a close look at these patterns, recognize the purpose they serve, and find alternatives.

There are good days and not-so-good days for us all. Welcome flexibility into your life so that when bumps in the road appear, you won't hear a fixed mindset telling you, "See! Failure! I knew this was going to happen. Why did I even try? It's not worth it!"

Instead, a growth mindset takes a deep breath and becomes curious. Curiosity creates resilience to handle challenges when they invariably appear. The growth mindset thinks, "Hmm, that didn't work as expected. Let's think about this. How could I have been better prepared? What support did I need that was lacking? Or was it just an unavoidable bump in the road?"

## Addressing urges and cravings

Habits are actions that have been repeated so many times that they become unconscious. We don't analyze them; we may not think about them at all. Can you remember back when you were learning to drive? Learning each and every step just to drive a few blocks took a lot of mental energy. Now for most of us, it's so ingrained, it's pretty much automatic. Going through the motions. It is the same with all habits. Given enough time and repetition, all habits become an unconscious series of actions.

Those unconscious actions may be working for or against you. If your habit is to get up first thing in the morning and meditate, practice yoga, or go for a run, that sounds like a healthy habit. If the unconscious habit, however, is to reach for a cigarette or whiskey at the first sign of stress, then that habit may not be the most supportive to your health. It is the very best coping mechanism your unconscious mind came up with to deal with the trigger (in this case stress), but it still may be worth addressing for long term health.

Create curiosity around your craving. Note it, become interested in it. Allow space for it. Do not immediately judge it, nor automatically indulge it. Instead, take a breath, look at it, and become curious.

Urges and cravings can be amplified by times of high stress, or not meeting our basic needs for sleep, water, food, connection, and comfort.

Is there a need not being taken care of when this habit arises? Invite reflection and curiosity. Think, journal, contemplate. For example, a sugar craving can have many sources, such as being stressed, lack of sleep, stopping your exercise routine, dehydration, undereating or relationship tension. Sometimes it's just a desire to eat sweets, but very often there is another trigger underlying the craving.

A few ways to interject a pause between the triggering feeling and the now not-so-automatic habit are:

- Practice mindfulness and redirection
- Go for a walk

- Inject a humorous break like watching a comedy show
- Drink a glass of water
- Have a high protein/fat snack

After giving yourself space and time for curiosity and reflection, check in with yourself after 20 minutes. What is the urge like now? Same? More or less intense? Has it transformed into feeling like another need?

This is an evolving process and just the tip of the iceberg in rooting out and changing behavioral patterns. I hope this has given you an initial insight into how to investigate habits you may want to change.

Changing your lifestyle will invariably change relationship dynamics between yourself and those close to you. While some changes may be good, some can be challenging. When you are making major lifestyle changes, it can help to share the reason for your change with those closest to you. Share your "why" with your support network—what is prompting you to make this desirable change. That way, they can more easily support you through your process, and be fully on board with your new plan.

Check in with yourself prior to planning big shifts in daily routines. Are you in a good place to tackle all this? Anxiety, depression, or other mental health concerns can, of course, create their own set of challenges. If this is relevant to you, I encourage you to first prioritize feeling stable with respect to your mental health (using the tools and care team you need) prior to attempting any big lifestyle, nutrition, or exercise changes—particularly if they are a radical shift from your current norm.

Additional key factors influencing your joint healing and recovery speed are sleep, stress, and connection.

Most of our time healing and regenerating new tissue happens while we sleep. Many people say that they can "get away" with five to six hours of sleep a night. However, barely functioning is not the same as getting the proper amount of sleep in order to heal. Over the long term, few can function optimally averaging only five to six hours of sleep a night. Most need seven to eight hours and some need nine to ten hours.

If sleep is a low priority for you (the "I'll sleep when I'm dead" mindset), I'll let Matthew Walker convince you of its utmost importance. His book *Why We Sleep*[27] details why we all need to prioritize sleep if we want a long and healthy life. Chronic pain and chronic under-sleeping is a bad combination.

If you are always cutting corners with late nights, early mornings, and living in a state of perpetual sleep deprivation, you are doing yourself a disservice as you will heal much slower.

High stress is another important factor, an epidemic in our society. Stress is not only associated with conditions such as anxiety and insomnia. Stress levels also play an important role in our joint health.

Stress triggers the release of "fight or flight" neurotransmitters such as adrenaline and hormones such as cortisol (often called the "stress hormone"). While these are necessary responses to get us out of grave danger, a constant flood of these stress reactions day in and day out take their toll.

Elevated cortisol is associated with cartilage degradation, bone spur formation,[28] and more severe osteoarthritis and joint pain.[29] Long-term high stress accelerates osteoarthritis, meaning an earlier diagnosis and more severe case if you are in a constant state of high stress.

Some forms of stress relief can provide double-duty when it comes to our 7 Step Plan. For example, most forms of exercise also improve stress levels. Calming physical activities such as restorative yoga, Tai Chi, or Qi Gong will be a better fit than a "power" fitness class if stress reduction is a goal of yours.

Your community is also an integral aspect of your health. This includes your friends, family, any group you share a close connection with. Having a strong team of support helps people live longer, better and with less pain.[30] Community really is medicine! So, take your daily dose by cultivating close, positive relationships.

Motivational speaker Jim Rohn is credited with saying that you are a product of the five closest people in your life. But is this really true? The answer is yes, and then some. Those influencing you and your health does not stop with the five people closest to you. Collectively, the health habits of all our friends— and even friends of friends you don't even know—influence the likelihood that we will follow suit whether that is body mass index,[31] smoking,[32] or happiness.[33]

So, take a look around and inventory your circle of friends and loved ones. The values and priorities of your group as a whole will reflect that which you also hold most dear. Where does health and happiness rank?

Those around you can provide inspiration or discouragement for your own health self-improvement. Value your time and energy. Choose wisely who gets access to it. If you need more positive influences in your circle, look to build relationships where you have common values, such as at a fitness class (valuing physical health and activity), or meditation group (valuing a healthy mindset).

Lastly, I need to address the few habits out there that will be working against you at every step to younger joints. We're talking tobacco and alcohol.

I'm not your middle-school health teacher, so I'm not here to lecture everyone about how "smoking is bad." I'm sure you've heard that countless times before, so let's skip it. I'm a physician who addresses chronic joint pain, so that's what we're talking about.

Regular use of tobacco products doesn't just harm your lungs. Tobacco use is associated with the development of knee osteoarthritis,[34] degenerative joint disease of the spine,[35] and degenerative disc disease.[36] Tobacco use damages all musculoskeletal tissue, from joints and spinal discs to muscles, tendons, cartilage, ligaments,[37] and bone,[38] If you experience chronic joint pain and currently smoke, make a plan to quit as one step in the right direction of taking care of and healing your joints.

Looking at research analyzing alcohol intake and arthritis is difficult, for a few reasons. One is that many studies are based on survey data, which asks research participants about their alcohol intake. Very few are tracking the effects of alcohol intake over time. The downsides of survey data are that some research participants may not want to reveal their true alcohol intake. Others may mark "no alcohol intake" because they cannot drink because of medications they are taking (for other chronic diseases) or are abstaining due to a history of alcohol abuse. Simply assessing joint health in those who do and do not drink alcohol is fraught with issues. However, we do see that alcohol has a greater association with osteoarthritis in women compared to men.[39]

We know that alcohol is dehydrating to joint tissue. Its effect is "dose-dependent." This means drinking two servings of alcohol per week is much less likely to trigger joint disease via dehydration than 14 servings a week. That may sound like a lot, but that's an average of just two drinks a day, slightly higher than the US average consumption of 9.5 drinks per week.

When it came to Jan, our plan focused first on addressing her alcohol intake. It was not uncommon for her to have two or three drinks on a typical day, and frequently up to four or five when socializing. She did not identify as having an addiction and did not feel it negatively impacting her life. It just was a part of her daily life.

Like so many others, it was the most convenient and easily accessed "tool" to decompress from work, as well as to address stress, anxiety or boredom. Her alcohol intake was normalized by her work and social environment. Though she had wanted to cut back for years, there had never been a compelling enough reason to do so before. Our treatment plan was an experiment to see how her hip pain responded to a reduction in her alcohol intake.

By methodically working through the key points in this chapter, we identified the thought patterns, triggers and current tools that ultimately were working against her. We then introduced new habits and patterns that were realistic, approachable, appealing and effective in supporting her creation and maintenance of positive health changes.

Over the course of two to three months, she cut down to an average alcohol intake of two servings on weekends. Most weekdays she remained alcohol free. Through this time, she slowly noticed her hip pain improving, along with other benefits of significantly reducing her alcohol intake, such as better sleep, energy, and less face puffiness. She was so happy to be free of the daily nagging hip pain that she ran up and bear hugged me when I saw her at that three-month follow up visit. I do tend to get a lot of hugs from patients after helping them eliminate their joint pain. It comes with the territory.

Our lifestyle habits can be our greatest asset or those which are most working against us. It takes intention and time, but we all have the capacity to heal and change. It starts with mindset. Further recommended reading on behavioral change and mindset is listed in the Younger Joints Today Toolkit at www.drcortal.com/toolkit.

STEP 1: Know Your Diagnosis

STEP 2: Eat to Heal Your Joints

STEP 3: Move and Strengthen Your Joints for Recovery

STEP 4: Address Lifestyle Factors

The Joint Gist

- Your habits matter- all of them.
- Habits can be changed, but not if they remain unconscious.
- Lifestyle factors that most impact joint health are sleep (are you getting your eight hours?), stress, social interaction, and alcohol and tobacco intake.

# STEP 5: Get Your Hormones in Check

I first met Stacy in the fall of 2018. Stacy is someone that anyone can get along with; friendly, kind, with a great sense of humor. We instantly hit it off and I was happy she came to see me for her chronic knee pain.

She had been having knee pain for years, maybe decades (sometimes it's hard to remember exactly when the pain started). Since turning 50 a few years back, the pain had become unbearable. She drove trucks for a living, which meant she was hopping in and out of the cab all day long. Or more accurately, in recent years she felt like she was crawling in and out of the driver's seat.

A recent spill out of the cab left her hobbling. She had landed with her full weight on her right kneecap, slamming right into the steps she used for getting into the truck.

An X-ray showed moderate osteoarthritis in both knees with chondromalacia patella (degenerative joint disease behind the kneecap) of the right knee.

She had heard about platelet-rich plasma injections (PRP), and came to me eager to get started with regenerative injection therapy to address her knee pain. However, during our first visit it was apparent there was more going on. In addition to her knee pain, she was also experiencing increased fatigue, she felt foggy-headed much of the time, muscle weakness, vaginal dryness and had zero sex drive. All of these symptoms had appeared over the last few years since her menstrual cycles stopped.

It was clear we needed to dig deeper. Instead of beginning with PRP injections, I suggested we first run a few tests, since she hadn't had any labs run in years. Most of the test results, such as blood sugar and thyroid levels, looked good. Her hormone panel was a different story. It showed low estrogen, her and testosterone was virtually nonexistent. It was a fraction of what we expected. I was suspicious that her hormone deficiencies were connected to her joint pain.

In this book on reversing joint pain, I am dedicating a whole chapter to hormones. This is not by accident. Hormones are that important to joint health. This is not just my opinion. This is established in and supported by research, as you will soon see. It's just that the dots are often not connected, or worse . . . entirely disregarded.

By the end of this chapter, I hope you will see how vital adequate hormone levels are for joint regeneration. If it is relevant to your case, I encourage you to discuss this with your healthcare provider.

The hormones of the greatest importance for us are insulin (first covered in Step 2 and briefly revisited here), thyroid, estrogen, and testosterone.

Hormones are messengers in our body that circulate and directly impact metabolic function of all our cells, tissues, and organs. They are vital for communication throughout our whole body.

### Insulin

Insulin is a hormone produced in the pancreas, which regulates blood glucose levels. Glucose is a simple sugar produced by the digestion of carbohydrates. It is a primary energy source for cells.

When it comes to insulin with respect to arthritis, the problem is generally too much. There are diseases associated with too little insulin (such as type 1 diabetes), but for the vast majority of those with insulin issues, it's a matter of excess.

Metabolic diseases affect a majority of US adults. This includes but is not limited to cardiovascular diseases, type 2 diabetes, pre-diabetes, elevated cholesterol, elevated triglycerides, abdominal obesity, and high blood pressure. In order to impact the course of these conditions, we must find and address the underlying factors of their development and progression.

What does any of this have to do with osteoarthritis? Well, one of the major dysfunctions underlying those metabolic diseases is insulin resistance. Insulin resistance is not one specific diagnosis; it is a hormonal imbalance that sets off many types of metabolic disease.

Insulin resistance involves excess production of insulin, as well as a decreased efficiency in its communication among the bloodstream and cells.

When someone with insulin resistance eats a typical meal, the carbohydrates (and proteins to a lesser extent) signal an overproduction of and inefficient use of insulin. The excess insulin must go somewhere, and one of the "spill over" locations is the joints. Insulin is very inflammatory and irritating to joints.[40]

I recommend patients get their blood sugar (glucose) and three-month blood sugar average (hemoglobin A1c) checked during their annual lab work, or perhaps more frequently if they are addressing metabolic disease.

Reversing insulin resistance is possible, as we've discussed in Step 2. I work with patients all the time to address this, but it first must be identified in order to be changed.

## Thyroid

For the most part, we are talking about hypothyroidism (too little thyroid hormone). Hyperthyroidism (too much thyroid hormone) can be a problem for our musculoskeletal system, causing accelerated bone loss (osteopenia and osteoporosis). But because hyperthyroidism comprises a small fraction of thyroid dysfunction (about 2-5%), we are focusing on hypothyroidism.

Your thyroid dictates many metabolic functions including your brain, hair, skin, nails, heart, digestive tract, fat cells, muscles, and joints. It's important for metabolism everywhere. When you do not produce enough thyroid hormone, or your body does not recognize and use it correctly, these systems can suffer.

Classic signs of hypothyroidism include fatigue, hair loss, weight gain and constipation. If you experience these, and have not had your thyroid checked recently, bring this up with your doctor. Even if you do not experience any of these symptoms, low thyroid function can still affect your musculoskeletal system. A few ill effects are onset or worsening of arthritis, fibromyalgia, and other chronic pain.

Thyroid levels are very closely linked to pain. Those with low thyroid function are more likely to experience more severe and widespread pain, earlier onset of joint degeneration, and worsened joint degenerative destruction.[41]

I have lost track of the number of times that—during the process of investigating a patient's chronic pain—we found and addressed their hypothyroidism. Without any other treatment, their pain significantly improved. Hypothyroidism hurts!

## Estrogen

Estrogen is important for tissue regeneration in women. Testosterone is as well. A decline in estrogen is often seen during perimenopause (around the time that menstrual periods stop), and for some comes with widespread effects. Along with the more commonly known symptoms such as hot flashes and night sweats, joint pain often accelerates during the menopausal shift. Declining estrogen is associated with the onset and worsening of osteoarthritis. This is seen as greater pain levels,[42] as well as earlier and more severe joint degeneration and cartilage loss.[43]

For perimenopausal and postmenopausal women, the hormone shifts can prompt arthritis and other degenerative changes in the spine. We can see this as spinal disc and facet joint degeneration.[44] Healthy joints and spines depend on adequate levels of estrogen to heal and prevent degeneration.

## Testosterone

Testosterone is another key hormone messenger that tells our body to build and regenerate, such as sites of injury and damage. Many are aware that testosterone builds muscle, but it also builds ligaments, tendons, and cartilage. Everyone needs adequate testosterone, not just men.

If you have a testosterone deficiency, your muscles, ligaments, tendons, and cartilage will repair and regenerate more slowly. They may also feel more painful.[45] Healing from past injuries may then take longer or heal incompletely.

Testosterone is important when it comes to arthritis. Because of its role in joint and connective tissue regeneration, low testosterone is associated with more severe osteoarthritis.[46]

As I had speculated, Stacy's hormone deficiencies were impacting her knee pain. Though she did have chronic knee pain for years, and did have a fall that worsened her pain and immobility, the estrogen and testosterone declining through menopause was what prevented her from healing as expected.

Within weeks of addressing her hormone deficiencies, she noticed significant improvement in her daily "aches and pains." Although we were happy with the response so far, her right knee pain (the one with chondromalacia patella) was still impacting her quality of life. At that point we decided to treat it with platelet-rich plasma injections (more on that in Step 7).

A month after completing two PRP sessions, she stopped noticing knee pain. It only ever bothered her if she really "pushed it" in the gym. I haven't seen her now in almost a year because she is doing great out happily living her life.

That's how I know I'm doing my job correctly. If we can identify the individual underlying causes to each person's joint pain, then I can truly address the them and help patients get better. "Graduating" patients from needing my care is the best part of my job.

Hormones help us heal. We need them to recover and build new tissue. When it comes to joints, healthy levels of hormones are necessary to regenerate muscle tissue, ligaments, tendons, and cartilage.

We touched on a few hormone deficiency symptoms in this chapter, and for more check out my *What Hormones?* Quiz available for my readers as part of the Younger Joints Today Toolkit at www.drcortal.com/toolkit.

If you are concerned about a hormonal deficiency, ask a doctor who specializes in this to evaluate you. Not every doctor who focuses on joint pain will be the best fit for hormone assessment and treatment, so be aware of this when you are putting together your care team.

STEP 1: Know Your Diagnosis

STEP 2: Eat to Heal Your Joints

STEP 3: Move and Strengthen Your Joints for Recovery

STEP 4: Address Lifestyle Factors

STEP 5: Get Your Hormones in Check

The Joint Gist

- We need hormones to heal.
- They are "Goldilocks" signals, not too much and not too little.
- Excess insulin drives joint pain.
- Deficiencies in thyroid, estrogen, and testosterone are important to address for joint pain.

# STEP 6: Supplements to Help Joints Heal

Supplements are just that: an addition to an already healthy diet and lifestyle. No number of supplements can make up for a poor diet and inactivity. After all the previous steps are in place, you can then look into supplementation for joint health.

What is your goal with supplementation? As you will see, some supplements are shown to be effective for pain relief, others for actual reversal of the osteoarthritis process. Depending on one's need, the supplements detailed below can assist with day-to-day pain levels or long term regression of degenerative change.[47]

For Rose, we were looking for both. At 72 years young, Rose has a spirit and energy to be envied by those half her age. I should know. Over the time I've known her, I've thought of her both as a role model for vibrant aging and as I jokingly remarked at one visit, my "spirit animal."

Rose is a go-getter. She is politically active, often out changing the world five days a week, sometimes every day of the week. Getting ballot signatures at the farmers market. Running booths for local, state, and national election campaigns. Her small stature might fool you, but she is an all-around dynamo. The only thing that was stopping her was her knee pain.

Over the past several decades her knee pain crept in slowly and was now interfering more and more in her daily life. She had to rest more often. She could only stand for about 30 minutes before the pain was unbearable. It was intruding upon activism and volunteering— and for energetic Rose this was simply unacceptable.

She needed to get back in action, and after reviewing all the prior five steps, we started with a supplementation trial.

## Collagen

As I've outlined in Step 2, collagen is a unique and vital building block of the musculoskeletal system. On a molecular level cartilage, ligaments, and tendons are comprised of mostly collagen fibers (50-98% depending on the exact tissue).

We see that providing this essential building block of healthy joint tissue improves joint pain.[48] Collagen supplementation is shown to increase collagen synthesis in cartilage tissue.[49] That is a good thing for those with osteoarthritis, since cartilage is primarily made of collagen fibers.

When choosing a collagen supplement, there are a few important factors to consider.

Since collagen is manufactured from animal products, the source counts. I don't want to be consuming supplements that come from factory feedlots. You can easily find a grass-fed or pastured collagen source (from cattle or pork).

Also, be aware of different forms of collagen. Collagen hydrolysate is a common form, and doesn't need to be cooked, unlike gelatin. Collagen powder can be easily mixed into water, coffee or another beverage.

If the package says gelatin, then it requires cooking. Jell-O is the most well-known example, but you can find plain gelatin in the store as well. I've included a few of my favorite homemade gelatin recipes in the appendix.

Lastly, there are sub-types of collagen available, such as types 1 and 3 (they always come together) and type 2. Many collagen supplements just say collagen hydrolysate and do not specify a type, so we presume they have them all.

Types 1 and 3 are concentrated in ligaments and tendon. If you are looking for building blocks for these specific tissues, they are most specific to that goal.

Type 2 collagen, on the other hand, is specifically concentrated in cartilage so may be more efficient for supporting cartilage healing (which is a major aspect of osteoarthritis). Significant improvement in pain levels using type 2 collagen have been seen at daily doses of 30-40 mg.[50]

Collagen supplementation as a whole proves to be useful in slowing cartilage degeneration and reducing joint pain.[51] Usual doses are one serving of gelatin (one tablespoon or seven grams of gelatin powder) or 30 grams of collagen hydrolysate.

Curcumin

Turmeric root has long been used as food and medicine in India. It contains curcuminoids which have wide-ranging effects on joint health, including reducing inflammation inside of joints and protecting cartilage cells from degeneration.[52] Tested against anti-inflammatory medication, curcuminoids at a dosage as little as 30 mg three times a day have been shown to be as effective at reducing joint inflammation as diclofenac sodium (a common NSAID medication).[53] This is great news because diclofenac can accelerate joint disease with long-term use.[54] Similar positive results have also been shown comparing curcumin to 1,200 mg per day of ibuprofen.[55]

As with collagen, not all curcumin supplements are created equal. Curcumin on its own has poor bioavailability in its natural form, so little gets absorbed from the digestive tract (and thus to the rest of the body, including the joints). To address this, various formulations exist, including some with high tech-sounding names like polymeric micelles and nanoparticles. These differ from a simple curcumin extract in that they are broken down into very small particles (nanoparticles) or are formulated with fatty acids (forming micelle compounds). The goal of all these formulations are to improve absorption.

Bioavailable curcumin at as little as 180 mg per day has been shown to not only significantly improve joint pain, and also help those who rely on other prescription or over the counter NSAIDs to reduce their reliance on these medications.[56]

### Essential Fatty Acids

As we've already touched on in Step 2, essential fatty acids such as monounsaturated fatty acids (MUFAs) and polyunsaturated fatty acids (PUFAs) are important for hormone and joint health. We can obtain these from foods or supplements.

You can get your daily dose of MUFAs by regularly incorporating minimally refined oils such as olive oil and sesame oil. These help lower inflammation associated with arthritis.[57] PUFAs have proven that they can slow down cartilage degeneration,[58] so both are important to regularly include in your diet.

Omega-3 fatty acids are one type of PUFA and have unique properties such as stimulating collagen synthesis and slowing down cartilage degrading enzyme activity.[59] These are important actions to support if you are trying to address osteoarthritis.

Omega-3 fatty acids are found in foods such as walnuts, flaxseeds, wild-caught salmon and grass-fed beef.[60] If you are not consuming foods high in MUFAs and PUFAs on a daily basis, supplementation can help make up this deficit.

Supplements are often derived from fish oil. Daily doses as little as 0.45 mg have been found to be effective for joint pain[61] (a 3-oz serving of salmon or sardines meets this dosage), though doses in the range of 1,000-2,000 mg are more commonly researched and used.[62] Lastly, Omega-3 fatty acids may have a synergistic effect with glucosamine. Some see the best effect when combining these supplements.[63]

### Glucosamine

There are many supplements on the market that contain glucosamine, so be aware of form and quality differences.

First, look at the last term used on a glucosamine supplement bottle. It will usually say glucosamine sulfate or glucosamine HCl. Glucosamine *sulfate* has the best evidence for supporting osteoarthritis. A few of these beneficial effects are stimulating cartilage formation,[64] improving joint pain and mobility, reducing pain,[65] and reducing arthritis progression. The typical dose in trials and used clinically is 500 mg three times a day.

There are also important factors with respect to glucosamine sulfate manufacturing. Look at the fine print of the supplement you have or are considering purchasing. I avoid those containing magnesium stearate in the "other ingredients" section.

This isn't the same as a magnesium supplement; it is an ingredient used in manufacturing. Since it appears to inhibit glucosamine absorption, I prefer brands that use leucine for this purpose instead.

When it came to Rose, I first carefully analyzed the long list of supplements she had been taking prior to starting care with me. After I reviewing the types, forms, other ingredients, and reasons she was taking them, I recommended she stop most of them and start taking glucosamine sulfate.

After starting the glucosamine, week by week she started to notice improvement. She could stand longer, now an hour at a time comfortably. It was easier to get up and down from her chair. She was not as stiff and achy in the morning.

Over the following months she continued to improve, and most recently reported that her knees are not stopping her at all. Rose has regained her former activism glory and we could not be more pleased.

As a parting note on supplementation, consult your doctor prior to starting any new supplement. Many supplements have interactions with medications (such as curcumin and blood-thinning medications), or other supplements you may be taking. These are research-backed supplements commonly used in my practice, but like every other step in this book, needs to be individualized to your unique needs.

Information and research on this topic is constantly changing. Specific products and manufacturers I know and trust are kept up-to-date in the Younger Joints Today toolkit at www.drcortal.com/toolkit.

STEP 1: Know Your Diagnosis

STEP 2: Eat to Heal Your Joints

STEP 3: Move and Strengthen Your Joints for Recovery

STEP 4: Address Lifestyle Factors

STEP 5: Get Your Hormones in Check

STEP 6: Supplements to Help Joints Heal

The Joint Gist

- Supplements can be helpful, but I am rarely relying solely on them to reverse joint pain.
- Supplements are finishing touches to a comprehensive plan.
- Glucosamine and curcumin have proven to be helpful for joint pain relief.
- Collagen and essential fatty acids have been shown to reverse arthritic changes in degenerating cartilage.

# STEP 7: Regenerative Injection Therapies – the latest in regenerative medicine

It's time to come back to my story. In the introduction, I detailed my injury, surgery and long and slow recovery. That even a decade post-injury, my knee was still weak, unstable, with episodes of pain. Perhaps you can relate.

Deciding to take my joint health in my own hands, I made a plan to reverse its trajectory, which over the years has become refined as my 7 Step Plan to Younger Joints Today. It all starts with getting a good diagnosis, and getting your nutrition, physical activity, lifestyle, hormones, and supplements in order.

After all that, then it can be the time to figure out whether you're a candidate for further treatment—whether that is regenerative injection therapies (RIT) or for some, surgery. No matter the type of interventions, they will be more successful if all the prior steps are first addressed.

That is the reason why RIT is saved for the very last step in our 7 Step Plan. To have an optimal response to this type of treatment, first get all the previous steps dialed in. Otherwise the injection may have minimal or no effect.

The RIT field is exploding in popularity and research. These injection therapies are a new take on an old problem, namely stimulating the body to heal chronic degeneration and injuries.

They work by an effect called stem cell migration. The injection provides key communication to the right spot. That is why getting the correct type of injection to the correct location is so important.

In essence they trick the body, causing a re-initiation of the healing cascade that is present within us all. If you've ever observed a cut or a swollen sprain heal, you have watched the healing cascade operate in real time.

The injections have several novel effects, beyond pain relief and inflammation reduction. In the case of osteoarthritis, there are studies showing a regeneration of cartilage tissue.[66] Each type of RIT has demonstrated positive results for joint pain and healing. Outlined below are the specific research findings for each.

In the orthopedic and sports medicine field, RIT is used to treat many types of connective tissue pathology, such as chronic injury and/or pain in ligament, tendon, cartilage, joint capsule, or meniscus tissue. Let's get into some specifics on what they are and when they are used.

### The many styles of regenerative injection therapies

### Prolotherapy

Prolotherapy was the first RIT on the scene and was first researched and widely written about by Dr. George Hackett, including his book published in 1958[67] and his many research articles published in that era. He was an orthopedic surgeon who treated thousands of patients in the 1950s and found that he could accelerate tissue healing (mostly ligament injuries) by injecting certain solutions into these sites of chronic injury. By experimentation with animals, and then later using the injections with his patients, he found that specific concentrations of solutions in certain connective tissue and joint sites could reliably produce pain-reversing and healing effects in joints and ligaments.

Over the following decades, there have now been hundreds of prolotherapy studies, looking at many types of chronic joint pain. Before we dive in, a brief word about research terminology.

Research results can be described as level 1 or level 2, on down to level 5. This is called the hierarchy of research. Level 1 results are considered the strongest evidence. This usually indicates multiple randomized controlled trials and/or systematic reviews or meta-analyses have found the same results. Levels 4 and 5 include case studies and expert opinions.

Evidence may also be described with an alphabetic rating, where A is strongest (comparable to level 1).

Prolotherapy has level 1 (or A) research results for use in knee osteoarthritis, rotator cuff injury, tennis elbow (lateral epicondylitis), and myofascial pain.[68] It has Level 2 (or B) research results in low back pain, osteoarthritis of other joints besides the knee, sacroiliac joint dysfunction, and many more conditions.[69]

Many prolotherapy studies follow participants over months or even years. Most studies show a notable reduction in pain (such as a 2014 study showing sustained improvement in knee pain a year later)[70] with minimal side effects. Research confirms what I see in office, which is that most patients are happy with the response (one systematic review of prolotherapy studies found patient satisfaction rates at 82%)[71] and that these effects usually remain for at least a year or longer after treatment.[72]

Prolotherapy has been used longer and is more widespread compared to the following RIT types. Though prolotherapy has the most extensive track record, this is not to say that it is better. They all have their best uses.

For one person with pain and instability of a partial rotator cuff tear or hip osteoarthritis, platelet-rich plasma injections may be the best fit. For another with pain from chronic sacroiliitis, prolotherapy may be the best fit. Discuss your unique needs with an injection expert if you are considering RIT, to find the right fit for you.

Platelet Rich Plasma

A few decades after prolotherapy's development, platelet-rich plasma (PRP) injections enter the scene. The 1990s saw an expansion of development and research of PRP for many orthopedic and sports medicine concerns. Some typical reasons for treatment are chronic pain, degenerative joint disease, and sports injuries.

As you may have guessed by the name, PRP is derived from a patient's own blood (via blood draw), then platelets and growth factors are concentrated from that sample. This concentrated plasma is then injected where healing is needed, such as in a joint affected by osteoarthritis.

The Level 1 research findings using PRP have focused on knee and hip osteoarthritis.[73] If that sounds similar to prolotherapy, you are right. Regardless of which type of RIT being studied, much of the research in this field is looking at changes in pain as it relates to osteoarthritis and other musculoskeletal sources of chronic pain.

A meta-analysis of PRP research for knee osteoarthritis published this year pooled the responses of 1,248 research participants spanning 12 studies, followed 12 months post-injections. These results indicate that PRP injections reduce knee pain and the positive response remains even a year later.[74]

All RIT types are on a spectrum. For some cases, PRP may provide a stronger, more efficient effect and be the desired treatment. Others may be a better candidate for the less aggressive prolotherapy treatment.

### Stem cell and stem cell-derived

Now we get to the newest forms of RIT: bone marrow-extracted (bone marrow aspirate concentrate or BMAC) stem cell injections and biologic allographs.

As the name suggests, BMAC takes the stem cells from the bone marrow of a patient (usually the back side of their hip bone) and injects that in a manner similar to the other RIT styles. Research is continuing to expand on all the types of RIT, and early research on BMAC (several of which are Level 2 studies) is looking promising for its use in knee osteoarthritis.[75, 76]

Biologic allographs are sometimes also called stem cells, but more accurately we can describe them as biologic products coming from umbilical and amniotic tissue (donated by healthy mothers during delivery). The tissue is processed into a sterile injectable product by a laboratory company specially outfitted to process them, then shipped to the RIT provider.

Though it has been found that by and large, these biologic injectable products available on the market (as of this writing) do not appear to contain live stem cells, research published this year shows that they do contain growth factors, extracellular vesicles, hyaluronic acid, and other compounds that can potentially be helpful for joint regeneration.[77]

Animal studies recently published have shown positive effects in cartilage growth.[78] Research participant trials are happening right now, looking at using biologic allograph injections for knee and hip osteoarthritis.

To look up ongoing research on this topic, search specific allograph product names at clinicaltrials.gov. One example is the company Surgenex. In 2018 I began following their study on human amniotic membrane injections for knee osteoarthritis. I saw on clinicaltrials.gob that it was recently completed and I expect to see the published article at any time. It will be fascinating to see how this field emerges and evolves.

One question I hope research will continue to investigate is whether and by how much biologic allographs and BMAC are superior to prolotherapy and PRP. For the latter two, level 1 research has been well established. In the coming years, we will see what research shows us in the stem cell injection realm.

So which injection is best for you? Like any treatment, it should be seen as a tool which needs to be customized to the right job.

Any potential injection procedure benefit must be weighed alongside its potential risk and downside, such as pain, adverse effects, invasiveness, and cost. There are other factors to consider as well, such as medical history and medications. This is all to say that not everyone is a candidate for RIT.

There is a good reason I have waited to Step 7 to discuss these. RIT relies on one's own body to heal, so all the other steps need to be addressed for it to properly work.

Since RIT relies on one's vitality, or ability to respond and heal, its ideal use is as part of a comprehensive approach to joint pain rather than as a stand-alone "miracle cure."

If someone's health is overburdened with inflammation, chronic diseases, hormone deficiencies or poor nutrition, their body cannot respond to the injections as well. They may not respond at all.

Using RIT in conjunction with good nutrition, movement practice, and a healthy lifestyle is an entirely different situation than with poor nutrition, inactivity, high stress, and sleep deprivation. The latter just will not respond well. The effect will be minimal in comparison and the injection can seem to be wasted, or at least significantly hindered.

It is worth spending a little time "tuning up the system," by considering all of the earlier steps to improve your health in a holistic and comprehensive manner.

My own path to healing involved an initial course of two prolotherapy sessions and one PRP session to my knee. I was then able to get to a radically different place with respect to my knee pain, function, and mobility.

I thought I'd have a crunchy, weak, unhappy knee my whole life . . . I was wrong.

I went from barely able to do a lunge pose to heavy weight lifting. It wasn't an overnight miracle—the process takes time—but RIT was a key piece of my healing. I am now closing my fourth decade of life with much better health and strength than I had when I was 20.

Any occasional prolotherapy or PRP I get now is to address minor injuries or overuse strains. It's now fine-tuning rather than bringing me back from the brink of disability like before.

It is on this happy note I conclude my 7 Step Plan. The final chapter will summarize how I put this all together, what to do when you feel stuck and where you can DIY versus when to get professional help.

STEP 1: Know Your Diagnosis

STEP 2: Eat to Heal Your Joints

STEP 3: Move and Strengthen Your Joints for Recovery

STEP 4: Address Lifestyle Factors

STEP 5: Get Your Hormones in Check

STEP 6: Supplements to Help Joints Heal

STEP 7: Regenerative Injection Therapies as the last step

The Joint Gist

- Regenerative injection therapies help by prompting healing where they are injected.
- There are different types, and they all have their benefits and drawbacks.
- Prolotherapy and PRP have been the most extensively researched, primarily focused on osteoarthritis.
- If you decide to get any RIT, take a look at all of the earlier steps in order to optimize your response to injection therapy.

# Putting it all together:

# where do we go from here?

Why is this all on your shoulders? Because it is very difficult to reverse a chronic health condition in our current medical system. It is set up more to manage conditions than heal them.

It comes down to a matter of different goals. If you seek care for joint pain, usually the goal is for you to stop complaining about joint pain. End of story.

No matter if you stop complaining because the pain-killing medication is dampening regeneration (such as cartilage healing pathways),[79] numbing the brain to nerve impulses, or any of the other mechanisms by which pain medication works. The task is to stop pain, so the goal is met.

The question is, what's your goal?

If your goal is to improve your health by looking at the whole picture, taking into consideration your unique reasons for joint degeneration, well . . . our current healthcare system just isn't set up well to address that.

As an example of just one of the steps in this book, you go to your rheumatologist for your joint pain and your endocrinologist for your hormone deficiency (if one is ever looked for, yet alone found). Each field of medicine is focused on its specialty. Hormones are not typically brought up in a rheumatology or pain medicine appointment.

The fact is, most of the steps in this book are generally disregarded in our standard of care model for joint pain. There may be no time for a comprehensive physical exam. Nutrition is often ignored, exercise is brushed off and you may be told hormones have nothing to do with your joints.

Our medical system is designed to look under a microscope, find one discrete pathology, and match a medication to it (or procedure or surgery) to make it go away.

That can work well for urgent and emergency medical needs. But for chronic conditions, many are left feeling like they have fallen through the cracks of the one-medicine-for-one-condition approach. When it comes down to it, we're complex biologic systems and multi-systemic health imbalances are not uncommon.

I'm not telling you to ditch your doctor. Please keep checking in, and getting your recommended labs and annual physical exams. However, if your chronic joint pain is not being adequately addressed by the standard of care approach (usually ibuprofen and physical therapy), then know that other options exist.

Beyond the standard model lies a comprehensive approach to identifying and addressing deficiencies and imbalances. It may just be what you need to get out of a rut and on your path to healing joint pain.

I'm not holding my breath that anytime soon the steps in this book will become the standard of care for addressing osteoarthritis, though I wish that were the case. I've written this book because this information needs to get out now. We can't wait until the entire medical establishment gets on board, since we know it takes an average of 17 years for research findings to become accepted in medical practice.[80]

The problem is, I didn't have time for that, my patients don't have time for that and I'm guessing that you don't either. Most of the research citations in this book are recent, many from just the last few years. Let's use the knowledge we have now to make changes starting today.

That's why this 7 Step Plan to Younger Joints Today exists. I want you to know of this evidence-informed framework and understand the treatment and interventions available to us today.

This approach is multidisciplinary, comprehensive, and spans the whole health of a person— top to bottom. It cannot be simplified down into one pill which is why I have my doubts about it getting adopted any time soon as the standard of care for osteoarthritis.

The important message here is that we all have an amazing capacity to heal, and that includes you!

Sometimes we encounter roadblocks, speed bumps, or other impediments on our road to recovery. That's ok. It's to be expected, so plan for it. When you've been living day in and day out with chronic, nagging joint pain, the path to healing is a process. It's often not one simple answer and rarely is an overnight turn-around. The path often involves ups as well as downs.

Celebrate the ups and make a game plan to address the downs. As long as the overall trajectory is going in the right direction, you're likely still on the right path.

With this 7 Step Plan, you can begin to take your health into your own hands and work proactively to improve your joint health. Let's take one last look at the whole 7 Step Plan for Younger Joints Today.

STEP 1: Know Your Diagnosis

STEP 2: Eat to Heal Your Joints

STEP 3: Move and Strengthen Your Joints for Recovery

STEP 4: Address Lifestyle Factors

STEP 5: Get Your Hormones in Check

STEP 6: Supplements Can Help Joints Heal

STEP 7: Regenerative Injection Therapies as the last step

Looking back over it all, where is the biggest gap in your current health picture?

If you have not gotten a comprehensive physical exam, then stop the presses and start with Step 1. The number of patients in chronic pain I have seen who say they have never had any physical exam *at all* is both alarming and heart-breaking. We have to know what is really going on in order to individualize a quality treatment approach.

How is your current diet? If your typical meals follow what we call the standard American diet, they may be loaded with sugary processed cereals and pastries for breakfast, followed by more refined carbohydrate-heavy meals centering around bread, pasta, rice, corn and other refined grains. While an insulin sensitive teenager can often get away with that diet, as the decades add up, most of the rest of us can't. This is particularly the case for those with osteoarthritis. Our joints require us to be as metabolically healthy as possible. If your meals tend to rely on quick, processed foods, use the nutrition information in Step 2 (and the shopping list, meal plans and recipes in the Toolkit at www.drcortal.com/toolkit) as a guide.

How is your activity level? If you are sedentary, get started with Step 3 and incorporate regular activity you enjoy. It could be walking your dog or a gentle yoga class. In the beginning, the most important thing is just to get (more) active.

Are alcohol, high stress, and sleep deprivation a part of your normal daily routine? If so, look over Step 4 and start to incorporate more lifestyle medicine changes to improve your joint health.

If you have been told you have a hormone deficiency or your answers to the *What Hormones?* Quiz in the Younger Joints Today Toolkit make you suspicious of one, take Step 5 to heart and talk with a hormone-savvy healthcare practitioner.

Are you ignoring all the other "less glamorous" steps and jumping right into supplements or injections? I hope now, equipped with all I've shared, you can step back and evaluate the whole picture. Regenerative injection therapies can often feel like, "Finally! This is magic!" But that's only if it's the right fit for the right candidate. Before you spend hundreds (or thousands) of dollars pursuing this type of care, do yourself a favor and make sure you have the other health foundations in place.

Are you confused by the number of supplement options out there, not sure which of the thousands of online options to pick from? Take a look at Step 6 to read about those with the strongest evidence backing, which are also those that I most frequently use in practice.

Lastly, if you've heard about prolotherapy, platelet-rich plasma, or stem cell injections and wonder if they're right for you, I hope that Step 7 has given you a jumping off point for learning what they are, when they are used and why.

After years of formulating this 7 Step Plan, this is the framework that I have determined works best. It is not necessary to address every step for every case, but at least consider whether it is relevant for you.

Some of these invariably require some type of professional evaluation, but most of the "heavy lifting," the actual day-to-day prioritization and attention, is done by us patients. My 7 Step Plan to Younger Joints Today is all the information I wish those out there experiencing chronic joint pain knew. I want to shout it from the rooftops!

It doesn't have to be this way.

You can be proactive.

You can heal.

My hope is that you have found value and insight in these previous pages. It is my goal for you to now fully understand, as I do, the real story about what we are all told is a permanent, unchangeable condition. One where the common refrain is that you must watch and wait until it eventually becomes "bad enough" to require surgery.

I hope to encourage you to seek out the type of care you deserve and get to a new place of health, strength, and movement. Just know that whenever you feel stuck, us joint pain experts are here to help you, every step of the way.

Your journey is your own. None of our journeys are exactly the same. I hope you now have some insight into how your path to joint health recovery can look. Starting today!

The Joint Gist

- If the standard approach isn't working for you, you're not alone.
- All our paths are unique; though consider every step.
- Much of the work really is up to you, though I hope it's supported by a caring health team.
- You can start today!

# Acknowledgements

First and foremost, I must show my heartfelt gratitude to my husband Xavi, who used his decades of kitchen experience in helping me craft our recipe chapter. He also graciously put up with my sudden inspirations of writing all hours of the mornings, nights and weekends.

I also could not have pulled this all together without the support and hard work of my editors Johanna Petronella Leigh and Dr. Caressa Gullikson, graphic design by Desi McAnally, photography by Kristal Passy and illustrations by Warren Muzak. In addition, I could not have done this without the support of numerous friends, family, and colleagues who have been there every step of the way, cheering me on to the publishing finish line.

I started writing this book when I realized I needed the word to get out to the world. That it's not too late. You're not "too far gone."

This information is the missing key that so many millions of Americans do not hear. Instead of waiting around for months and years until the pain is so bad that you're finally "bad enough" for a joint replacement surgery, there are proactive steps you can take. Now.

You can heal. I believe it because I see it every day in office.

Use this book as a tool to guide your next steps forward. What has not been evaluated for you? What has not been brought up? A five minute appointment will not cover everything in this book, so you may have to look beyond that model. I hope this has given you hope and ideas in taking your next steps.

This book has been a labor of love—something that required tireless hours of work to completion—between juggling my clinical practice (which had its own upending transition during our pandemic and quarantine changes) and practicing what I preach by incorporating all the steps I have shared each day in my life—such as weight lifting, nutrition, stress reduction, sleep, and the occasional regenerative injection therapy.

If you have enjoyed this book, if you have learned something new, please leave me a review on Amazon. My whole goal is to spread the word to others living with chronic joint pain that healing is possible, and I need your help and support to make that possible. I wish you the best on your road to Younger Joints Today.

Dr. Angela Cortal is a Naturopathic Physician based in Oregon. She is passionate about reversing degenerative joint disease by addressing the root causes. She loves partnering with her patient to optimize their health, happiness, strength, and well-being.

In addition to her clinical practice, she is a sought-after teacher focusing on addressing joint pain, instructs advanced injection skill courses for physicians, and lectures to professional audiences (on hormones, joint health, and injection therapies). In her spare time she tends her rural property with her husband Xavi and their two rescue dogs, Levi and Frankie.

You can find out more at www.drcortal.com.

# Appendix

## Recipes

First a quick note

All of these recipes have been tested many times in our kitchen and in kitchens of our close friends and family.  Many recipes did not make the cut. Below are those that did.

Each recipe will indicate whether it provides adequate sources of protein, fat and/or collagen.  All are important to include as a regular part of your daily diet.

Deciding what to include here and what to cut was a months-long struggle. You won't find recipes on how to scramble eggs, cook a burger, or grill a steak.  Those are all great basics to know, but that's not what I'm focusing on here. Ultimately I decided to include those recipes that are very valuable to the nutrition of your joints but that you may not readily find elsewhere. Some are a new twist on a common recipe.

For my Canadian and other international readers: I'm sorry the US does not use the metric system.  It would make all our lives a lot easier if we did. Instead of bogging the recipes down with writing multiple measuring systems here, the recipes here are using US standard teaspoons, tablespoons, cups, etc. since that is what I am used to.  Since a tablespoon for you is as useless as telling me how many grams of butter to use, you will find a metric version of all these recipes in the Younger Joints Today Toolkit at www.drcortal.com/toolkit.

## Breakfast

### Easy Almond Flour Pound Cake

Protein-rich          Healthy Fats

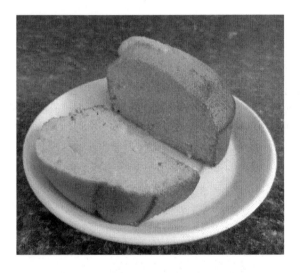

Servings: 4 (two 4-inch springform pans*)

Prep time: 5-10 minutes

Cook time: 40-50 minutes

Ingredients:

¼ cup plus 2 tbsp Butter

2 cups almond flour

4 extra-large eggs (or 6 medium eggs)

1 tbsp pure bourbon vanilla extract

½ cup monk fruit sweetener

½ tsp salt

Directions:

Preheat oven to 350°F.

Line bottom of springform pans with parchment paper, generously grease the inner sides and bottom of the springform pans with butter.

Melt ¼ c butter (on stove or microwave) but avoid boiling it.

Add almond flour, eggs, salt and the monk fruit sweetener into stand mixer or mix by hand in mixing bowl. Add in the vanilla extract and slowly pour in the melted butter. It should look like a batter consistency (like cake batter) when thoroughly mixed.

Spoon the batter into the springform pans, filling to the top. It is fine if the batter mounds over the top.

Place the spring form pans on a baking sheet for easy handling and place on middle rack of oven.

Bake for approximately 45 minutes or until an inserted toothpick comes out clean.

Cut into 2 or 4 pieces and serve by itself with coffee, or topped with butter, cheese (slices of mild cheddar, gouda or cream cheese) or your own desired toppings.

Additional flavoring ideas include adding in a zest of a half lemon, ¼ tsp cinnamon or ½ tsp "pumpkin pie spices."


*If you do not have 4" springform pans, you may want to consider getting yourself a pair so you can make mini cakes. Mini cakes are fun to make. But as a substitute, you can use either a standard loaf pan (8-1/2 x 4-1/2 x 2-1/2 inches) and add 5 minutes cook time, or a muffin pan and subtract 5 minutes cook time.

# Super Energy Nut & Seed Granola

Protein-rich          Healthy Fats

Servings: 4 cups

Prep time: 15 minutes

Cook time: 20 minutes

Ingredients:

2 eggs, separated

½ cup monk fruit powder

2 tbsp butter, softened

1 tbsp salt

½ cup almond butter

1 tbsp vanilla extract

2 tbsp blanched almond flour

2 tbsp flax seed meal

1 tbsp cinnamon

1 cup pumpkin seeds, raw and shelled

1 cup sunflower seeds, raw and shelled

1 cup hemp seeds, hulled

2 cup nuts, raw and roughly chopped.  Whatever nuts you prefer: one type or a mixture.  Walnuts, pecans, almonds, hazelnuts, pistachios

and/or brazil nuts will work.

Directions:

Preheat oven to 300°F.

In a stand mixer with the flat beater (or mixing bowl), add in the egg whites, monk fruit powder and butter. Save the yolks for another recipe (see "Impress your friends" Key Lime Pie parfait below).

Mix until the butter is well incorporated. Add in the salt, almond butter and vanilla extract and continue mixing. Then add in the almond flour, flax seed meal and cinnamon. Stop mixing when all is well incorporated.

Next add in the pumpkin, sunflower seeds and hemp seeds.

Your nuts should be small-ish. If they are already chopped or slivered that will work. Otherwise chop them down to small pieces and add into the mixture. Mix until all nuts are lightly coated and it will all start clumping together and now is starting to look like granola.

Crumble the granola mixture onto a nonstick baking sheet and bake in oven for 15 minutes, then turn all the granola over with a pancake turner or spatula so that you cook both sides. Bake for another 15 minutes, then remove from the oven and let cool.

With your granola cooling on the counter, flip over the granola again with a spatula to release more moisture. Let it cool down completely before storing, as this will make it most crunchy. Once it is room temperature, it is ready to serve or store.

Some serving ideas include: full-fat Greek yogurt, coconut cream (thicker than coconut milk) or unsweetened nut milk if you are looking for more of a cereal-and-milk alternative.

Store at room temp in a clean, dry glass jar and use it up within a week.

If you're feeling fancy, use the granola as the base for the "Impress your friends" Key Lime Pie parfait below.

## Blueberry Muffins with Cream Cheese

Protein-rich                    Healthy Fats

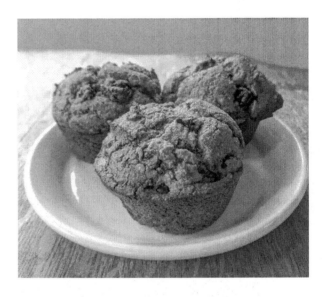

Servings: 12 muffins

Prep time: 15 minutes

Cook time: 35 minutes


Ingredients:

½ cup butter (plus 1 tbsp if not using cupcake liners), softened

2/3 cup monk fruit sweetener powder

1 tsp. salt

2 eggs

1 cup almond flour

1 ½ cup green banana flour

1 tbsp. baking powder

1 tbsp. flax seed meal

1 cup whole milk yogurt

2 cups frozen blueberries

1 tbsp pure bourbon vanilla extract

Cream cheese to top

Directions:

Preheat the oven to 350°F. Either use cupcake liners or grease the muffin pans with melted butter to prevent sticking.

In a medium mixing bowl add the almond flour, green banana flour and baking powder and stir until it's all combined.

In a stand mixer, add the eggs, butter, monk fruit sweetener and salt (or mix by hand in separate mixing bowl) until well incorporated. Add the yogurt and vanilla extract to the wet mix and continue mixing.

Put the dry mix into the wet mix and keep mixing. When it looks like a cake batter consistency, drop in the frozen blueberries and continue mixing a just a few more moments until the blueberries are dispersed.

Scoop the muffin batter into the pan using two large spoons (or an ice cream scooper* if you have one), distributing evenly among the sections. Set in center rack of the oven and bake for about 35 minutes, until an inserted toothpick comes out clean.

Set on a baking rack to cool then top with cream cheese.

* You can get away with not having an ice cream scoop, but they are very handy in the kitchen for controlling portions of all types of

mixtures.  These (or cookie scoops which are very similar) have a spring-loaded thumb trigger for popping out your mixture.  They come in many sizes and I find the 2 oz and 5 oz most handy.  We use ours all the time for meatballs and baked goods.

Shakshuka – aka Poached Eggs in (Delicious) Tomato Sauce

Protein-rich          Healthy Fats

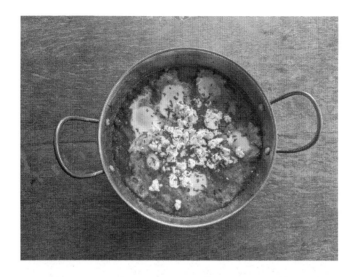

You can find many variations on this dish from North Africa, Egypt, Israel and other parts of the Middle East. Here is our brunch-ready adaptation.

Servings: 4

Prep time: 15 minutes

Cook time: 35 minutes


Ingredients:

3 tbsp olive oil

1 large onion (white or yellow), chopped

1 large red bell pepper, chopped

½ tsp salt

3 cloves garlic, minced

3 tbsp tomato paste

1 tsp ground cumin

½ tsp smoked paprika

¼ tsp red pepper flakes (if you want the heat)

1 large can (28 oz) crushed tomatoes, fire-roasted if you can find it

Black pepper, freshly ground to taste

6 medium eggs

5 oz feta, crumbled

2 tblsp flat-leaf parsley, chopped


Directions:

Preheat the oven to 375°F.

Warm up the olive oil over medium heat in a large stainless steel skillet. This is one of the times I favor stainless steel over cast iron on the stove, to save your cast iron's seasoning and avoid imparting an acrid taste.

Add the onion and bell pepper, cooking until they are soft. Next add in the garlic, tomato paste, cumin, paprika and red pepper flakes. Stir for a minute or two.

Then add in the tomatoes, stirring a little and bringing it just up to a simmer. Keep it simmering for another 10 minutes, until it starts thickening. Add in the salt and pepper, adjusting to taste.

Now comes the fun part, making nests for the eggs. One at a time, create a depression with the back of a large spoon and crack an egg inside the depression. Spoon a little bit of the sauce up and over the edges of the whites to keep each egg in place. Work around the skillet until you have nested each egg. Sprinkle a bit of salt and pepper on top of each egg.

Finish by baking the skillet in the oven for about 15 minutes. You are looking for the egg whites to turn opaque and the egg yolks to look risen and soft. Shakshuka eggs are traditionally a little runny, but you can cook it a few extra minutes if you like your eggs firm.

Remove the skillet from the oven - careful, it's heavy and hot! Garnish with the feta and parsley then scoop up and enjoy.

## "What's in the Fridge" Truita

Protein-rich          Healthy Fats

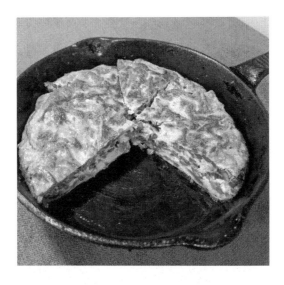

A truita is also called a Spanish omelet. Truita is a Catalan version of an eggs-and-things-omelet.  It's not a classic American omelet, this is more like a baked egg dish.  You can serve this for any meal.  The slices also pack great; you can serve warm or room temperature.

Servings: 6

Prep time: 15 min

Cook time: 20 min

Ingredients:

¼ cup olive oil

1/3 cup red onion, sliced

2 cups of vegetables … what's in the fridge?

Options: 1 bunch asparagus (the thinner the better). Trim the ends (snap off the thick woody parts) and cut into thirds.

You can use any vegetable you would sauté such as broccoli, kale, zucchini or peppers.

3 button mushrooms, sliced

½ cup diced meat, such as ham, prosciutto or other cured meat

6 eggs

1 ½ tsp salt

1 tsp black pepper, ground


Directions:

Crack the eggs in a small mixing bowl and whisk to an even consistency. Set aside.


Use a 6" cast iron pan* on the stove top and use medium heat to sweat down onions in oil. Lightly fry them until they turn a light golden color (they will become translucent). Then add in the sliced mushrooms and cook until they brown. Add in asparagus (or whatever veggies you are using), and cook until they soften and get darker in color.

Don't add salt during the frying stage, or the whole thing will get too wet.

Transfer the veggie mix to a medium mixing bowl and let rest for 2 minutes then add in the whisked eggs (we rest them so they don't cook the eggs right away). Now add in the salt, pepper and diced meat.

Add 1 tbsp olive oil back into the (now empty) cast iron pan and set to /medium-low heat. Then add the egg, veggie and meat mixture back into the pan.

After 1-2 minutes, use a fork to work all around the whole eggy edge, slightly lifting it away from the edge of the pan. This builds up its crust.

Cook for another 5 minutes, then take the fork and check the edges to see if they are loose. Is the truita loose or is it stuck to the pan? We want it to be loose. Try jiggling the pan to see if the truita is loose.

Now it's time to flip it. Don't worry, we'll walk through this together. I believe in you.

This is not a pancake flip maneuver, you won't be throwing anything up in the air.

Get a dinner plate that is larger than your pan. Hold the plate in your non-dominant hand. Pick up the cast iron pan with your other hand (using a handle guard or mitt).

Walk everything over to your sink (liquid egg is sneaky and can escape). Turn the plate upside-down and place it like a lid on the pan, completely covering the cast iron pan. Put your non-dominant hand on top of the plate, essentially pinning the plate between you and the pan. Rotate it all 180 degrees, flipping it over so now the truita has plopped down onto your plate and your pan is now upside-down and empty.

Way to go, kitchen pro!

Add one more tbsp of olive oil into the pan, then slide the truita back into the pan so we can cook the formerly-top-now-bottom of the dish. After 5 minutes, remove from heat and set on a plate to cool.

Cut into 6 wedges. You can garnish with finely sliced green onions or a sprinkle of cheese, but we usually just eat it as is.

* If you don't have a 6" cast iron pan, you can use one larger or smaller, that will just change the thickness of your truita.  If you don't have any cast iron pans, you could use a nonstick pan (use a saucepan with vertical walls rather than frying pan with sloping walls). I really don't trust the chemicals used in nonstick pan technology, so just get yourself a cast iron pan, learn to season it, and thank me later.

Lunch & Dinner


"Kitchen Sink" Bone Broth


Collagen-rich


I wasn't sure where this recipe fit, since bone broth is a great base for many soups, sauces and other savory items, so lunch & dinner it is.

Bone broth is one of those recipes that's easy and versatile.
You can find bone broth in just about any grocery store, but after learning this recipe you'll see it's simple and very inexpensive to make it yourself.

It's also a great way to add collagen to your diet.


Servings: 4 (2 quarts)

Prep time: 10 minutes

Cook time: 25 hours


Ingredients:

1 white or yellow onions, chopped

1 head of celery, chopped

1 clove of garlic (up to 6, depending on how much you like garlic)

1 bunch of parsley, chopped

2 tbsp apple cider vinegar

2 tsp salt

3-4 quarts water

2 pounds of bones, whatever you have saved on hand. Just about any bones left over from cooking bone-in meat will work. A few ideas are oxtail, marrow bones, short ribs, shanks and chicken carcasses. If you're buying bones specific for this, pork knuckles and chicken feet may be the most reasonably priced. We keep a container in our freezer just for leftover bones, and add to it until we have enough for a batch.

Directions:

First roast the bones in the oven at 400°F for 30 minutes. Toss those bones into an 8 quart stock pot (see below for slow cooker option) and deglaze your roasting pan with a little water.

Add in the vinegar. Add in at least 3 quarts of water, enough to entirely cover the bones but still allow room in the pot for the water to boil. Set to high heat. Once boiling, turn down to the lowest simmer possible and cover with the lid slightly ajar.

Simmer for 12 hours. Check on it occasionally, skimming off any foam as it appears.

Add in the onions, celery and parsley and simmer for another 12 hours.* Add the garlic in and let simmer for one last hour.

When your broth is done it will have a very rich, deep color and savory smell. Adjust salt to taste.

Set a fine-mesh strainer on top of a large bowl to strain your broth, to separate bone and vegetable pieces.

Cool using an ice bath in the sink, or refrigerate in small containers. I like freezing some of the bone broth in ice cube trays so that I have small portions to use in soups, sauces or just to warm up in a mug.

Depending on the fat content of your meat bones, you may have a large or small layer of fat coagulate on top of your broth when it cools. I save that for other recipes.

Slow cooker: Using the recipe above, first set to High to start simmering the broth, then set to Low for the remainder of the cooking. Be sure to check your settings, to see if your High gets hot enough and if your Low is low enough for a low simmer. If you have a smart electric pressure cooker (i.e. Instant Pot), you can use it for both the roasting and bone broth simmering steps.

* Yes that adds up to a day-plus cooking time, but I don't expect you to stay up overnight cooking. If simmering bone broth on your back burner isn't safe for your kitchen, the crock pot or Instant Pot would be your next easiest options. Otherwise cooking, cooling, then cooking again the following day would be your last workaround.

# Mediterranean Salad

Protein-rich          Healthy Fats

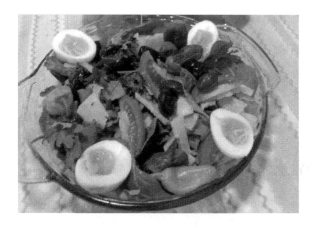

This Mediterranean Salad is more of an ad-libs salad, "throw a little bit of what you have on hand together," than an actual recipe. There are specifics below, of course, but I really invite you to experiment and come up with delicious new combinations in your home.

Servings: 4

Prep time: 15 minutes


Salad Ingredients:

1 small head of lettuce, I prefer red-leaf or oak

½ small red onion, peeled and sliced

½ English cucumber, sliced

½ cup red bell pepper, diced – raw or roasted

½ cup tomatoes (I prefer cherry tomatoes), chopped

½ cup olives (I prefer Arbequina or the Trader Joe's Marinated olive duo – see my shopping list in the Toolkit)

1 4-6 oz tin canned fish preserved in non-canola oil (rather than water) such as sardines in sunflower oil, mackerel in sunflower oil or tuna in olive oil

2 eggs, boiled and halved

½ cup feta cheese, crumbled or parmesan cheese, sliced


Dressing Ingredients:

2 tbsp olive oil

2 tbsp red wine vinegar

½ tsp salt

½ tsp black pepper

That's it. That's the basis of most of my salad dressings. Those four sit on my dining room table, always at the read for a salad.

If you want to make a fancier vinaigrette, some options include (any or all):

1 tsp. Dijon mustard

1 tsp oregano, dried

1 tsp thyme, dried


Directions:

Assemble the salad, top with the dressing and enjoy. Watch out if your olives have pits!

This is a very flexible salad. It is ok to leave out a vegetable if you don't have it, and add another as it suits you (you can see the pepperoncini in the photo above; our salads change a little every time).

Try different meats. Try different cheeses- or omitting them if you prefer. So long as you have lettuce, onion, tomato, some sort of meat or other protein and the four dressing ingredients, then you're off to a solid start. There are even some Mediterranean salad versions that don't have the lettuce at all. Experiment and find out what you like best.

Protein-rich               Healthy Fats               Collagen-rich

Confit is a slow cook method where it's entirely submerged under oil while cooking. The result is very tender, rich, flavorful meat that has many uses. You can eat it simply with sautéed veggies, stuff it in a baked pepper or use it to top really anything where you want super moist comfort-food-level meat.

A little also goes a long way, due to this cooking method. Baked or grilled, I would probably eat two or three chicken thighs at a typical mea, but confit style I'm feeling full after one (maybe one and a half on a weight lifting day).

Servings: 4

Prep time: 15 minutes (not counting overnight seasoning)

Cook time: 13 hours (in a crockpot)

Ingredients:

4 chicken thighs, bone-in, skin on

6 garlic cloves, peeled and pounded

3 bay leaves

3 cups mushrooms, sliced (can be buttons, a mushroom mix or your preference)

¼ cup poultry seasoning

Salt, enough to coat chicken plus 1 tsp

½ yellow or white onion, diced

3 cups sunflower oil (yes, this takes a lot of oil)

Directions:

Generously salt the thighs, then sprinkle with 2 tbsp poultry seasoning and garlic powder. Place in a dish with a lid in the fridge for at least 8 hours (up to 24 hours for more flavor). The next day, rinse them off and pat them dry with a paper towel.

Place them in a crockpot with the garlic, bay leaves, mushrooms, 1 tbsp poultry seasoning and 1 tsp salt.

Pour enough oil on top that you entirely cover the chicken, vegetables and spices plus another ½ inch for good measure.

Set the crockpot to high until it reaches 180°F, then turn it down to warm (or the lowest setting) and cook 12 more hours.

Serving options include eating it right away, searing the thighs or keeping it in the fridge* to add to later meals.

To sear the thighs, add ¼ c. of the oil to a hot skillet, then place the thighs in skin side down until crispy.

* A note about storage: the confit will last a very long time in the fridge (several weeks at least) if after the 12 hour slow cook, you transfer all your meat and veggies to another container (preferably ceramic or glass) and cover it all with the warm oil. Place in the fridge. When it cools the congealed oil creates a gel top that preserves the meat.

**Oxtail soup**

Protein-rich          Healthy Fats          Collagen-rich

This is one of the highest collagen soups I have found. You will see just how much collagen your soup contains when you reheat it after being refrigerated. The entire soup will be one big gelled block, or a collagenous porridge-like consistency.

Servings: 4

Prep time: 15 minutes

Cook time: 3.5-4.5 hours

Ingredients:

1/3 cup bacon fat

5 lbs oxtails (about 6 large oxtails)

1 medium onion, coarsely chopped

1 large carrot, peeled and coarsely chopped

2 sticks celery, coarsely chopped

3 cloves of garlic, coarsely chopped

1 turnip, peeled and coarsely chopped

1 gallon water

3 bay leaves

Salt, to taste

Directions:

Over high heat on your stovetop, heat up the bacon fat in a large stock pot, then add the oxtails.

Brown the oxtails on both sides then remove them from the pot.

Turn the burner down to medium-high then sweat down the chopped onion (cook it until it turns translucent).

Next add the carrot and celery and cook until they start to brown. Add the garlic, cook for one more minute then add the water. Scrape around the walls and bottom of the pot so nothing sticks.

Now add the oxtails back in and the bay leaves at this time.

Let it all come up to boil, then turn the heat down to low and simmer until oxtails get soft (about 3-4 hours). You know it's done cooking when the oxtails have softened (squeeze them with tongs to check).

At this point add salt to taste, and put in your chopped turnip.

Cook for 15 more minutes then remove from heat and serve warm. This is a fork-and-spoon soup. You'll want the form to remove the meat from the bones.

Snacks

Deviled eggs

Protein-rich                    Healthy Fats

Servings 4 (yields 12 deviled eggs)

Prep time: 5 minutes

Cook time: 25 minutes

Ingredients:

6 medium eggs

4 slices bacon

1-2 heaping tbsp mayo (store-bought or see the Quick Homemade Mayo recipe)

1/2 tsp salt

1 tsp lemon juice

1 green onion, sliced

Directions:

Place the bacon on a baking sheet and bake at 350°F for 15-20 minutes until they start to look lightly cooked but are still soft (not yet crispy). Turn the oven off and drain off the fat (which we save for other recipes). Put the bacon back in the oven (it's still off) and let it sit for another 10 minutes. Drain off the rest of the fat.

While you are waiting for the bacon, put the eggs in a saucepan and fill with enough water to cover them by an inch. Boil the eggs on the stove over medium-high heat for 6-7 minutes. Drain off the hot water, then add cold tap water and ice cubes to rapidly cool them.

Peel the eggs, cut them in half and scoop out yolks.

Add the yolks and bacon in the food processor* (use the chopper blade) and pulse until diced consistency. Add the mayo, salt, lemon juice and green onion then continue to process until fairly smooth. You will still see little flecks of bacon and onion, but it's not extremely lumpy.

Use two spoons to transfer the mixture to the egg halves. Use one spoon to scoop the filling out of the processor, and the other to direct the filling off that spoon and into the egg. Heap them up high.

Garnish with paprika, finishing salt (big flaky fancy salt you can buy in a gourmet grocery store) or just eat as is.


* You can of course mix the eggs and bacon by hand if you do not have a food processor, but it takes finely dicing the bacon and mashing the egg yolks to achieve a similar consistency.


**Dressings & Sauces**


Quick Homemade Mayo


Healthy Fats


Yield: 1.5 cups

Prep time: 5 minutes

Ingredients:

1 cup sunflower oil

1 x-large or jumbo egg (or 2 mediums)

1 tsp stoneground mustard

1 tbsp lemon juice

1/2 tsp salt

1/4 tsp garlic powder

1 tsp cider vinegar

Directions:

Combine all ingredients directly in a large mouth pint-sized mason jar. Blend with stick blender, starting at the bottom and moving up to incorporate all the oil until it has achieved a uniform thick consistency (about 1-2 minutes). Use the blender or a spatula to make sure any oil on the top of the mayo is well incorporated into the mix.

Both under-blending and over-blending can "break" the mayo (the egg and oil separate). Aim for the mayo to be thick and creamy with no slick oiliness on top.

If you don't have a stick blender (also called a hand blender or immersion blender) you can use a standard countertop blender if you have the "food stomper" attachment in the lid so that you can push the oil down into the mayo when blending.

Note: this recipe does contain uncooked egg in its end product. We personally source our eggs from local, pasture-raised farms, which are less prone to food-borne infection risks. It is ultimately your decision whether to consume these types of foods.

**Blue Cheese Dressing**

Healthy Fats

Yield: 2 cups

Prep time: 5 minutes

Ingredients:

1/2 cup mayo (homemade recipe above or store bought)

1/2 cup sour cream

2 oz blue cheese

1/4 tsp garlic powder

1/4 tsp onion granules

1/2 tsp coarse ground black pepper

1 tbsp fresh parsley, chopped

Directions:

Combine all ingredients in a stand mixer or mix by hand in a mixing bowl.

**Monk fruit BBQ sauce**

Actually, this one's just for fun

Yield: 2 cups

Prep time: 15 minutes

Cook time: 15 minutes

Ingredients:

1/2 cup bacon fat (saved from any of the previous recipes calling for cooked bacon)

1 small onion, chopped

4 cloves garlic, minced

1/4 cup chili powder

1 quart can diced tomatoes

1/2 cup apple cider vinegar

1 tsp nutmeg

Monk fruit sweetener powder, to taste

Salt, to taste

Directions:

On the stove top over medium-high heat, sweat down the onion in bacon fat until it begins to brown. Add in the garlic. When garlic begins to brown (only about a minute later), stir in the chili powder, then add the diced tomatoes.

Turn down to medium and continue cooking until the liquid in the pan has almost entirely cooked off. Then add in the apple cider vinegar and nutmeg.

Remove from the heat and allow to cool.

Now it's time to make this chunky sauce smooth. To filter out all the large chunks, pour the mixture through a food mill or sieve, whatever you have on hand. As an alternative, you can just blend it all up in a food processor with the S-blade attachment. This works fine though your sauce will end up orange instead of red, but tastes the same.

Add in salt and sweetener to taste (I like mine more savory and less sweet so I add about 1 tsp of salt and only about a ½ tsp of monk fruit sweetener).

Desserts


"Impress your friends" Key Lime Pie gelatin parfait

Collagen-rich

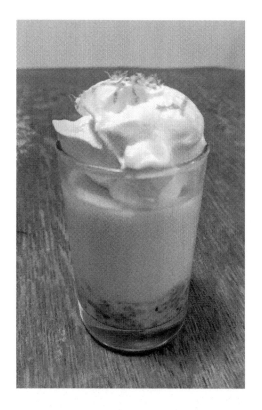

This one is as fun to serve as it is to eat.

Servings: 4

Prep time: 40 minutes

Cook time: 20 minutes

Parfait Crust Directions:

Make a batch of the Super Energy Nut & Seed Granola recipe above.

Press ¼ cup granola into the bottom of your four serving containers. We use 6 oz "juice glasses" (that are never actually used for juice), but any 6-8 oz glassware will work. Set aside while you make the gelatin filling.

Key Lime Pie Gelatin Filling:

Ingredients:

1 cup water

2 tsp gelatin (I prefer Great Lakes brand)

¼ cup monk fruit powder (white powder will be lighter colored, golden will be darker, but either works)

1 large lime, zest from the whole peel and juiced (3 oz)

½ cup heavy whipping cream

2 egg yolks

Directions:

In your measuring cup, pour the gelatin over the top of the water and stir it in with a spoon, mixing until the gelatin has dissolved into the water (that's called "blooming the gelatin").

In a medium saucepan on the stove, add the gelatin water and monk fruit powder. Turn up to medium heat, bringing to a boil. Stir occasionally.

While the gelatin is cooking, zest the lime and try to avoid zesting any pith (white part of the lime peel).

Cut the lime in half and squeeze out all the juice into a measuring cup and set aside.

Beat the heavy cream and egg yolks in a small bowl, just enough to incorporate in the egg yolks.

Let the gelatin boil lightly for a minute. At this point it should turn translucent.

Add in the lime juice and the cream to the egg mixture. Stir continuously to avoid curdling.

Bring it back up to a boil then remove from the heat. With the pan off the stove, add in ¾ of the lime zest to the pan (set aside the rest for garnish) and stir to incorporate.

After the gelatin has cooled and started to thicken (the consistency of condensed milk), pour the gelatin over the granola crust in the glasses, filling 2/3 full. Refrigerate for at least 1 hour.


Whipped Cream Topping:

½ cup heavy whipping cream

½ tsp vanilla extract

Monk fruit sweetener liquid extract (optional), 5 drops

Whisk cream and vanilla in a bowl until it makes stiff peaks.

Top the now-cooled gelatin with the whipped cream and sprinkle on the remaining lime zest.

# Bibliography

1.

Zhang, Yuqing, and Joanne M. Jordan. 2010. "Epidemiology of Osteoarthritis." *Clinics in Geriatric Medicine* 26, no. 3: 355–69. https://doi.org/10.1016/j.cger.2010.03.001.

2.

National Collaborating Centre for Chronic Conditions (UK). 2008. *Osteoarthritis: National Clinical Guideline for Care and Management in Adults (NICE).* Royal College of Physicians (UK).

3.

Kim, Chan, Michael C. Nevitt, Jingbo Niu, Mary M. Clancy, Nancy E. Lane, Thomas M. Link, Steven Vlad, et al. 2015a. "Association of Hip Pain with Radiographic Evidence of Hip Osteoarthritis: Diagnostic Test Study." *BMJ* 351 (December): h5983. https://doi.org/10.1136/bmj.h5983.

4.

Kijowski, Richard, Donna G. Blankenbaker, Paul T. Stanton, Jason P. Fine, and Arthur A. De Smet. 2006. "Radiographic Findings of Osteoarthritis versus Arthroscopic Findings of Articular Cartilage Degeneration in the Tibiofemoral Joint." *Radiology* 239, no. 3: 818–24. https://doi.org/10.1148/radiol.2393050584.

5.

National Center for Chronic Disease Prevention and Health Promotion (NCCDPHP). 2019. "Arthritis- How CDC Improves Quality of Life for People With Arthritis." Page last reviewed January 30, 2020. https://www.cdc.gov/chronicdisease/resources/publications/factsheets/arthritis.htm.

6.

Hootman, Jennifer M., and Charles G. Helmick. 2006. "Projections of US Prevalence of Arthritis and Associated Activity Limitations." *Arthritis and Rheumatism* 54, no. 1: 226–229. https://doi.org/10.1002/art.21562.

7.

National Cancer Institute (NCI). "Cancer Stat Facts: Cancer of Any Site." Accessed July 7, 2020. https://seer.cancer.gov/statfacts/html/all.html.

8.

American Diabetes Association. "Statistics About Diabetes." Accessed July 7, 2020. https://www.diabetes.org/resources/statistics/statistics-about-diabetes.

9.

Dingle, J. T. 1999. "The effects of NSAID on the matrix of human articular cartilages." *Zeitschrift für Rheumatologie* 58, no. 3: 125-129. https://doi.org/10.1007/s003930050161.

10.

Brinjikji, Waleed, Patrick H. Luetmer, Bryan Comstock, Brian W. Bresnahan, L. E. Chen, R. A. Deyo, Safwan Halabi et al. 2015. "Systematic Literature Review of Imaging Features of Spinal Degeneration in Asymptomatic Populations." *American Journal of Neuroradiology* 36, no. 4: 811–816. https://doi.org/10.3174/ajnr.A4173.

11.

Araújo, Joana, Jianwen Cai, and June Stevens. 2019. "Prevalence of Optimal Metabolic Health in American Adults: National Health and Nutrition Examination Survey 2009–2016." *Metabolic Syndrome and Related Disorders* 17, no. 1: 46–52. https://doi.org/10.1089/met.2018.0105.

12.

Rezaianzadeh, Abbas, Seyedeh-Mahdieh Namayandeh, and Seyed-Mahmood Sadr. 2012. "National Cholesterol Education Program Adult Treatment Panel III Versus International Diabetic Federation Definition of Metabolic Syndrome, Which One is Associated with Diabetes Mellitus and Coronary Artery Disease?" *International Journal of Preventive Medicine*, 3, no. 8: 552–558.

13.

Araújo, Joana, Jianwen Cai, and June Stevens. 2019. "Prevalence of Optimal Metabolic Health in American Adults: National Health and Nutrition Examination Survey 2009–2016." *Metabolic Syndrome and Related Disorders* 17, no. 1: 46–52. https://doi.org/10.1089/met.2018.0105.

14.

Rosillo, María Angeles, Marina Sánchez-Hidalgo, Alejandro González-Benjumea, José G. Fernández-Bolaños, Erik Lubberts, and Catalina Alarcón-de-la-Lastra. 2015. "Preventive effects of dietary hydroxytyrosol acetate, an extra virgin olive oil polyphenol in murine collagen-induced arthritis." *Molecular Nutrition and Food Research* 59, no. 12, 2537–2546. https://doi.org/10.1002/mnfr.201500304.

15.

McAfee, Alison J., E. M. McSorley, G. J. Cuskelly, A. M. Fearon, B. W. Moss, J. A. M. Beattie, J. M. W. Wallace, et al. 2011. "Red Meat from Animals Offered a Grass Diet Increases Plasma and Platelet n -3 PUFA in Healthy Consumers." *British Journal of Nutrition* 105, no. 1: 80–89. https://doi.org/10.1017/S0007114510003090.

16.

Baker, Kristin R., N. R. Matthan, A. H. Lichtenstein, Jingbo Niu, Ali Guermazi, Frank Roemer, Andrew Grainger et al. 2012. "Association of Plasma N-6 and n-3 Polyunsaturated Fatty Acids with Synovitis in the Knee: The MOST Study." *Osteoarthritis and Cartilage* 20, no. 5: 382–387. https://doi.org/10.1016/j.joca.2012.01.021.

17.

Isanejad, Masoud, Jaakko Mursu, Joonas Sirola, Heikki Kröger, Toni Rikkonen, Marjo Tuppurainen, and Arja T. Erkkilä. 2016. "Dietary Protein Intake Is Associated with Better Physical Function and Muscle Strength among Elderly Women." *British Journal of Nutrition* 115, no. 7: 1281–1291. https://doi.org/10.1017/S000711451600012X.

18.

Zwart, A. H. de, M. van der Leeden, L. D. Roorda, M. Visser, M. van der Esch, W. F. Lems, and J. Dekker. 2019. "Dietary Protein Intake and Upper Leg Muscle Strength in Subjects with Knee Osteoarthritis: Data from the Osteoarthritis Initiative." *Rheumatology International* 39, no. 2: 277–284. https://doi.org/10.1007/s00296-018-4223-x.

19.

Rizzoli, René, Emmanuel Biver, J-P. Bonjour, Veronique Coxam, D. Goltzman, J. A. Kanis, J. Lappe et al. 2018. "Benefits and Safety of Dietary Protein for Bone Health—an Expert Consensus Paper Endorsed by the European Society for Clinical and Economical Aspects of Osteopororosis, Osteoarthritis, and Musculoskeletal Diseases and by the

International Osteoporosis Foundation" *Osteoporosis International* 29, no. 9: 1933–1948. https://doi.org/10.1007/s00198-018-4534-5.

20.

    Zelfand, Erica. 2020. "Collagen Peptides." Posted February 1, 2020. https://archive.theamericanchiropractor.com/article/2020/2/1/collagen-peptides

21.

    Skelly, A. C., Roger Chou, Joseph R. Dettori, Judith A. Turner, Janna L. Friedly, Sean D. Rundell, Rongwei Fu, et al. 2020. "Noninvasive Nonpharmacological Treatment for Chronic Pain: A Systematic Review Update." *Agency for Healthcare Research and Quality (US)*. https://doi.org/10.23970/AHRQEPCCER209.

22.

    Zampogna, Biagio, Rocco Papalia, Giuseppe Francesco Papalia, Stefano Campi, Sebastiano Vasta, Ferruccio Vorini, Chiara Fossati, Guglielmo Torre, and Vincenzo Denaro. 2020. "The Role of Physical Activity as Conservative Treatment for Hip and Knee Osteoarthritis in Older People: A Systematic Review and Meta-Analysis." *Journal of Clinical Medicine* 9, no. 4: 1167. https://doi.org/10.3390/jcm9041167.

23.

    Vincent, Kevin R., and Heather K. Vincent. 2020. "Concentric and Eccentric Resistance Training Comparison on Physical Function and Functional Pain Outcomes in Knee Osteoarthritis." *American Journal of Physical Medicine and Rehabilitation* (April). https://doi.org/10.1097/PHM.0000000000001450.

24.

    Hurley, Ben F., and Stephen M. Roth. 2000. "Strength training in the elderly: Effects on risk factors for age-related diseases." *Sports Medicine* 30, no. 4: 249-268. https://doi.org/10.2165/00007256-200030040-00002.

25.

    Reeve IV, Thomas E., Timothy E. Craven, Matthew P. Goldman, Justin B. Hurie, Gabriela Velazquez-Ramirez, Matthew S. Edwards, and Matthew A. Corriere. 2020. "Outpatient Grip Strength Measurement Predicts Survival, Perioperative Adverse Events, and Non-Home Discharge among Patients with Vascular Disease." *Journal of Vascular Surgery* S0741-5214(20)31090-9. https://doi.org/10.1016/j.jvs.2020.03.060.

26.

Dweck, Carol S. 2007. *Mindset: The New Psychology of Success.* Random House Digital, Inc.

27.

*Walker, Matthew. 2017. Why We Sleep: Unlocking the Power of Sleep and Dreams. Simon and Schuster.*

28.

Hossain, Farhad Md., Yunkyung Hong, Yunho Jin, Jeonghyun Choi, and Yonggeun Hong. 2019. "Physiological and Pathological Role of Circadian Hormones in Osteoarthritis: Dose-Dependent or Time-Dependent?" *Journal of Clinical Medicine* 8, no. 9: 1415. https://doi.org/10.3390/jcm8091415.

29.

Carlesso, Lisa C., John A. Sturgeon, and Alex J. Zautra. 2016. "Exploring the Relationship between Disease-Related Pain and Cortisol Levels in Women with Osteoarthritis." *Osteoarthritis and Cartilage* 24, no. 12: 2048–2054. https://doi.org/10.1016/j.joca.2016.06.018.

30.

Cortal, Angela. 2020. "Social Connection: A Missing Piece of Your Treatment Plan?" Posted July 2, 2020. https://ndnr.com/pain-medicine/social-connection-a-missing-piece-of-your-treatment-plan/.

31.

Christakis, Nicholas A., and James H. Fowler. 2007. "The Spread of Obesity in a Large Social Network over 32 Years." *The New England Journal of Medicine* 357, no. 4: 370-379.

32.

Christakis, Nicholas A., and James H. Fowler. 2008. "The collective dynamics of smoking in a large social network." *The New England Journal of Medicine* 358, no. 21:2249-2258.

33.

Fowler, James H., and Nicholas A. Christakis. 2008. "Dynamic spread of happiness in a large social network: longitudinal analysis over 20 years in the Framingham Heart Study." *BMJ* 337:a2338. https://doi.org/10.1136/bmj.a2338.

34.

Venkatachalam, Jayaseelan, Murugan Natesan, Muthurajesh Eswaran, Abel K. Samuel Johnson, V. Bharath, and Zile Singh. 2018. "Prevalence of osteoarthritis of knee joint among adult population in a rural area of Kanchipuram District, Tamil Nadu." *Indian Journal of Public Health* 62, no. 2, 117–122. https://doi.org/10.4103/ijph.IJPH_344_16.

35.

Brotherson, Jason D., Elaine S. Marshall, Gary Measom, John R. Clark. 2003. "Tobacco use and degenerative joint disease of the spine." *Journal of the American Academy of Nurse Practitioners* 15, no. 6: 277-281. https://doi.org/10.1111/j.1745-7599.2003.tb00398.x.

36.

Steelman, Theodore, Louis Lewandowski, Melvin Helgeson, Kevin Wilson, Cara Olsen, and David Gwinn. 2018. "Population-based Risk Factors for the Development of Degenerative Disk Disease." *Clinical Spine Surgery* 31, no. 8: E409–E412. https://doi.org/10.1097/BSD.0000000000000682.

37.

Al-Bashaireh, Ahmad M., Linda G. Haddad, Michael Weaver, Debra Lynch Kelly, Xing Chengguo, and Saunjoo Yoon. 2018. "The Effect of Tobacco Smoking on Musculoskeletal Health: A Systematic Review." *Journal of Environmental and Public Health* 4184190. https://doi.org/10.1155/2018/4184190.

38.

Nasto, Luigi A., Kevin Ngo, Adriana S. Leme, Andria R. Robinson, Qing Dong, Peter Roughley, Arvydas Usas et al. 2014. "Investigating the role of DNA damage in tobacco smoking-induced spine degeneration." *Spine Journal* 14, no. 3: 416–423. https://doi.org/10.1016/j.spinee.2013.08.034.

39.

Takiguchi, Ryoya, Rintaro Komatsu, Kaori Kitamura, Yumi Watanabe, Akemi Takahashi, Ryosaku Kobayashi, Rieko Oshiki et al. 2019. "Modifiable factors associated with symptomatic knee osteoarthritis: The Murakami cohort study." *Maturitas* 128: 53-59. https://doi.org/10.1016/j.maturitas.2019.06.013.

40.

Kim, Hyeonkyeong, Donghyun Kang, Yongsik Cho, and Jin-Hong Kim. 2015. "Epigenetic regulation of chondrocyte catabolism and anabolism in osteoarthritis." *Molecules and Cells* 38, no. 8: 677-684. https://doi.org/10.14348/molcells.2015.0200.

41.

Voloshyna, L., O. Doholich, and I. Sithinska. 2017. "Hypothyroidism—a special comorbidity factor in patients with osteoarthrosis: clinical, pathophysiological and prognostic aspects." *Georgian Medical News* 272: 53-59.

42.

Wáng, Yì Xiáng J., Jùn-Qīng Wáng, and Zoltán Káplár. 2016. "Increased low back pain prevalence in females than in males after menopause age: evidences based on synthetic literature review." *Quantitative Imaging in Medicine and Surgery* 6, no. 2: 199. https://doi.org/10.21037/qims.2016.04.06.

43.

Wang, Yi Xiang J. 2017. "Menopause as a potential cause for higher prevalence of low back pain in women than in age-matched men." *Journal of Orthopaedic Translation* 8: 1-4. https://doi.org/10.1016/j.jot.2016.05.012.

44.

Wang, Yi-Xiang J., and James F. Griffith. 2011. "Menopause causes vertebral endplate degeneration and decrease in nutrient diffusion to the intervertebral discs." *Medical Hypotheses* 77, no. 1: 18-20. https://doi.org/10.1016/j.mehy.2011.03.014.

45.

Jin, X., B. H. Wang, X. Wang, B. Antony, Z. Zhu, W. Han, F. Cicuttini et al. 2017. "Associations between endogenous sex hormones and MRI structural changes in patients with symptomatic knee osteoarthritis." *Osteoarthritis and Cartilage* 25, no. 7: 1100-1106. https://doi.org/10.1016/j.joca.2017.01.015.

141

46.

Sowers, MaryFran, Marc Hochberg, Jeffrey P. Crabbe, Anthony Muhich, Mary Crutchfield, and Sharon Updike. 1996. "Association of bone mineral density and sex hormone levels with osteoarthritis of the hand and knee in premenopausal women." *American Journal of Epidemiology* 143, no. 1: 38-47. https://doi.org/10.1093/oxfordjournals.aje.a008655.

47.

Castrogiovanni, Paola, Francesca Maria Trovato, Carla Loreto, Houda Nsir, Marta Anna Szychlinska, and Giuseppe Musumeci. 2016. "Nutraceutical supplements in the management and prevention of osteoarthritis." *International Journal of Molecular Sciences* 17, no. 12: 2042. https://doi.org/10.3390/ijms17122042.

48.

Kumar, Suresh, Fumihito Sugihara, Keiji Suzuki, Naoki Inoue, and Sriraam Venkateswarathirukumara. 2015. "A double-blind, placebo-controlled, randomised, clinical study on the effectiveness of collagen peptide on osteoarthritis." *Journal of the Science of Food and Agriculture* 95, no. 4: 702-707. https://doi.org/10.1002/jsfa.6752.

49.

Vaishya, Raju, Amit Kumar Agarwal, Amish Shah, Vipul Vijay, and Abhishek Vaish. 2018. "Current status of top 10 nutraceuticals used for Knee Osteoarthritis in India." *Journal of Clinical Orthopaedics and Trauma* 9, no. 4: 338-348. https://doi.org/10.1016/j.jcot.2018.07.015.

50.

Lugo, James P., Zainulabedin M. Saiyed, and Nancy E. Lane. 2015. "Efficacy and tolerability of an undenatured type II collagen supplement in modulating knee osteoarthritis symptoms: a multicenter randomized, double-blind, placebo-controlled study." *Nutrition Journal* 15, no. 1: 14. https://doi.org/10.1186/s12937-016-0130-8.

51.

Juher, Teresa Figueres, and Esther Basés Pérez. 2015. "Revisión de los efectos beneficiosos de la ingesta de colágeno hidrolizado sobre la salud osteoarticular y el envejecimiento dérmico." *Nutrición Hospitalaria* 32, no. 1: 62-66. https://doi.org/10.3305/nh.2015.32.sup1.9482.

52.

Chin, Kok-Yong. 2016. "The spice for joint inflammation: anti-inflammatory role of curcumin in treating osteoarthritis." *Drug Design, Development and Therapy* 10: 3029. https://doi.org/10.2147/DDDT.S117432.


53.

Kertia, Nyoman, Ahmad H. Asdie, and Wasilah Rochmah. 2012. "Ability of curcuminoid compared to diclofenac sodium in reducing the secretion of cycloxygenase-2 enzyme by synovial fluid's monocytes of patients with osteoarthritis." *Acta Medica Indonesiana* 44, no. 2: 105-113.


54.

Reijman, Max, S. M. A. Bierma-Zeinstra, H. A. P. Pols, B. W. Koes, B. H. C. Stricker, and J. M. W. Hazes. 2005. "Is there an association between the use of different types of nonsteroidal antiinflammatory drugs and radiologic progression of osteoarthritis?: The rotterdam study." *Arthritis and Rheumatism* 52, no. 10: 3137-3142. https://doi.org/10.1002/art.21357.


55.

Kuptniratsaikul, Vilai, Piyapat Dajpratham, Wirat Taechaarpornkul, Montana Buntragulpoontawee, Pranee Lukkanapichonchut, Chirawan Chootip, Jittima Saengsuwan, et al. 2014. "Efficacy and safety of Curcuma domestica extracts compared with ibuprofen in patients with knee osteoarthritis: a multicenter study." *Clinical Interventions in Aging* 9: 451-458. https://doi.org/10.2147/CIA.S58535.


56.

Nakagawa, Yasuaki, Shogo Mukai, Shigeru Yamada, Masayuki Matsuoka, Eri Tarumi, Tadashi Hashimoto, Chieko Tamura, et al. 2014. "Short-term effects of highly-bioavailable curcumin for treating knee osteoarthritis: a randomized, double-blind, placebo-controlled prospective study." *Journal of Orthopaedic Science* 19, no. 6: 933-939. https://doi.org/10.1007/s00776-014-0633-0.


57.

Rosillo, María Angeles, Marina Sánchez-Hidalgo, A. González-Benjumea, José G. Fernández-Bolaños, Erik Lubberts, and Catalina Alarcón-de-la-Lastra. 2015. "Preventive effects of dietary hydroxytyrosol acetate, an extra virgin olive oil polyphenol in murine collagen-induced arthritis." *Molecular Nutrition and Food Research* 59, no. 12 2537-2546. https://doi.org/10.1002/mnfr.201500304.

58.

Baker, Kristin R., N.R. Matthan, A.H. Lichtenstein, Jingbo Niu, Ali Guermazi, Frank Roemer, Andrew Grainger, et al. 2012. "Association of Plasma N-6 and n-3 Polyunsaturated Fatty Acids with Synovitis in the Knee: The MOST Study." *Osteoarthritis and Cartilage* 20, no. 5: 382–387. https://doi.org/10.1016/j.joca.2012.01.021.

59.

Jerosch, Jörg. 2011. "Effects of glucosamine and chondroitin sulfate on cartilage metabolism in OA: outlook on other nutrient partners especially omega-3 fatty acids." *International Journal of Rheumatology* 969012. https://doi.org/10.1155/2011/969012.

60.

McAfee, Alison J., E. M. McSorley, G. J. Cuskelly, A. M. Fearon, B. W. Moss, J. A. M. Beattie, J. M. W. Wallace, et al. 2011. "Red Meat from Animals Offered a Grass Diet Increases Plasma and Platelet n -3 PUFA in Healthy Consumers." *British Journal of Nutrition* 105, no. 1: 80–89. https://doi.org/10.1017/S0007114510003090.

61.

Hill, Catherine L., Lynette M. March, Dawn Aitken, Susan E. Lester, Ruth Battersby, Kristen Hynes, Tanya Fedorova et al. 2016. "Fish oil in knee osteoarthritis: a randomised clinical trial of low dose versus high dose." *Annals of the Rheumatic Diseases* 75, no. 1: 23-29. https://doi.org/10.1136/annrheumdis-2014-207169.

62.

Peanpadungrat, Pornrawee. 2015. "Efficacy and safety of fish oil in treatment of knee osteoarthritis." *Journal of the Medical Association of Thailand* 98, Suppl 3 : S110-14.

63.

Gruenwald, Joerg, Ellen Petzold, Regina Busch, Heinz-Peter Petzold, and Hans-Joachim Graubaum. 2009. "Effect of glucosamine sulfate with or without omega-3 fatty acids in patients with osteoarthritis." *Advances in Therapy* 26, no. 9: 858-871. https://doi.org/10.1007/s12325-009-0060-3.

64.

Reginster, Jean-Yves. 2007. "The efficacy of glucosamine sulfate in osteoarthritis: financial and nonfinancial conflict of interest." *Arthritis and Rheumatism* 56, no. 7: 2105-2110. https://doi.org/10.1002/art.22852.

65.

Jerosch, Jörg. 2011. "Effects of glucosamine and chondroitin sulfate on cartilage metabolism in OA: outlook on other nutrient partners especially omega-3 fatty acids." *International Journal of Rheumatology* 969012. https://doi.org/10.1155/2011/969012

66.

Topol, Gastón Andrés, Leandro Ariel Podesta, Kenneth Dean Reeves, Marcia Mallma Giraldo, Lanny L. Johnson, Raul Grasso, Alexis Jamín, et al. 2016. "Chondrogenic effect of intra-articular hypertonic-dextrose (prolotherapy) in severe knee osteoarthritis." *PM&R* 8, no. 11: 1072-1082. https://doi.org/10.1016/j.pmrj.2016.03.008.

67.

Hackett, George S., G. A. Hemwall, and G. A. Montgomery. 1958. *Ligament and tendon relaxation*. Charles C. Thomas.

68.

Hauser, Ross A., Johanna B. Lackner, Danielle Steilen-Matias, and David K. Harris. 2016. "A systematic review of dextrose prolotherapy for chronic musculoskeletal pain." *Clinical Medicine Insights: Arthritis and Musculoskeletal Disorders* 9: 139-159. https://doi.org/10.4137/CMAMD.S39160.

69.

Rabago, David, Andrew Slattengren, and Aleksandra Zgierska. 2010. "Prolotherapy in primary care practice." *Primary Care: Clinics in Office Practice* 37, no. 1: 65-80. https://doi.org/10.1016/j.pop.2009.09.013.

70.

Rabago, David, Jeffrey J. Patterson, Marlon Mundt, Aleksandra Zgierska, Luke Fortney, Jessica Grettie, and Richard Kijowski. 2014. "Dextrose and morrhuate sodium injections (prolotherapy) for knee osteoarthritis: a prospective open-label trial." *The Journal of Alternative and Complementary Medicine* 20, no. 5: 383-391. https://doi.org/10.1089/acm.2013.0225.

71.

Hassan, Fadi, Suad Trebinjac, William D. Murrell, and Nicola Maffulli. 2017. "The effectiveness of prolotherapy in treating knee osteoarthritis in adults: a systematic review." *British Medical Bulletin* 122, no. 1: 91-108. https://doi.org/10.1093/bmb/ldx006.

72.

Rabago, David, Richard Kijowski, Michael Woods, Jeffrey J. Patterson, Marlon Mundt, Aleksandra Zgierska, Jessica Grettie, et al. 2013. "Association between disease-specific quality of life and magnetic resonance imaging outcomes in a clinical trial of prolotherapy for knee osteoarthritis." *Archives of Physical Medicine and Rehabilitation* 94, no. 11: 2075-2082. https://doi.org/10.1016/j.apmr.2013.06.025.

73.

Le, Adrian DK, Lawrence Enweze, Malcolm R. DeBaun, and Jason L. Dragoo. 2018. "Current clinical recommendations for use of platelet-rich plasma." *Current Reviews in Musculoskeletal Medicine* 11, no. 4: 624-634. https://doi.org/10.1007/s12178-018-9527-7.

74.

Hohmann, Erik, Kevin Tetsworth, and Vaida Glatt. 2020. "Is platelet-rich plasma effective for the treatment of knee osteoarthritis? A systematic review and meta-analysis of level 1 and 2 randomized controlled trials." *European Journal of Orthopaedic Surgery and Traumatology* 14 Feb, 2020: 1-13. https://doi.org/10.1007/s00590-020-02623-4.

75.

Shapiro, Shane A., Shari E. Kazmerchak, Michael G. Heckman, Abba C. Zubair, and Mary I. O'Connor. 2017. "A prospective, single-blind, placebo-controlled trial of bone marrow aspirate concentrate for knee osteoarthritis." *The American Journal of Sports Medicine* 45, no. 1: 82-90. https://doi.org/10.1177/0363546516662455.

76.

Chahla, Jorge, Chase S. Dean, Gilbert Moatshe, Cecilia Pascual-Garrido, Raphael Serra Cruz, and Robert F. LaPrade. 2016. "Concentrated bone marrow aspirate for the treatment of chondral injuries and osteoarthritis of the knee: a systematic review of outcomes." *Orthopaedic Journal of Sports Medicine* 4, no. 1: 2325967115625481. https://doi.org/10.1177/2325967115625481.

77.

Gupta, Ashim, Saadiq F. El-Amin, Howard J. Levy, Rebecca Sze-Tu, Sobrasua E. Ibim, and Nicola Maffulli. 2020. "Umbilical cord-derived Wharton's jelly for regenerative medicine applications." *Journal of Orthopaedic Surgery and Research* 15, no. 1: 1-9. https://doi.org/10.1186/s13018-020-1553-7.

78.

Cheng, Jai-Hong, Ching-Jen Wang, Wen-Yi Chou, Shan-Ling Hsu, Jen-Hung Chen, and Tsai-Chin Hsu. 2019. "Comparison efficacy of ESWT and Wharton's jelly mesenchymal stem cell in early osteoarthritis of rat knee." *American Journal of Translational Research* 11, no. 2: 586-598.

79.

Dingle, J. T. 1999. "The effects of NSAID on the matrix of human articular cartilages." *Zeitschrift für Rheumatologie* 58, no. 3: 125-129. https://doi.org/10.1007/s003930050161.

80.

Morris, Zoë Slote, Steven Wooding, and Jonathan Grant. 2011. "The answer is 17 years, what is the question: understanding time lags in translational research." *Journal of the Royal Society of Medicine* 104, no. 12: 510-520. https://doi.org/10.1258/jrsm.2011.110180.

Made in the USA
Las Vegas, NV
22 June 2021